Madame Chinchilla

STEWED, SCREWED AND TATTOOED is not just a phrase, it is an old ritual. Sailors long at sea looked forward to port stops to satisfy their cravings. STEWED obliterated the abstinence of being a sober and alert crew member. Getting SCREWED filled the void of a long period spent without the favors of a lady. And getting TATTOOED helped record the experience of the seafaring adventure.

STEWED, SCREWED AND TATTOOED does not neccessarly apply to all who desire a tattoo. Virgins (both sexes) get tattooed, teetotalers get tattooed, and those who have never been to sea get tattooed. Mankind has a deep primitive need to decorate himself both temporarily with attire, hairstyle, and jewelry and permanently with scarification, body modification and tattooing. This book reveals a cross-section of the various body decor of people of the earth, and also their cultures, motivations and desires to be adorned with symbols of their choice.

Captain Don Leslie
Sword Swallower and
Circus Side Show Attraction–1996

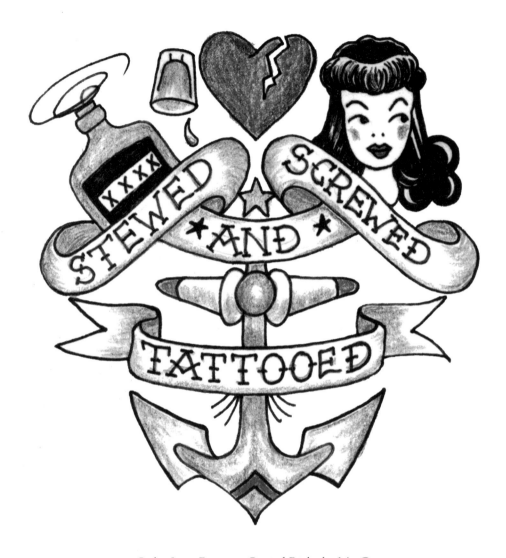

Sailor Jerry Design – Copied Right by Mr. G

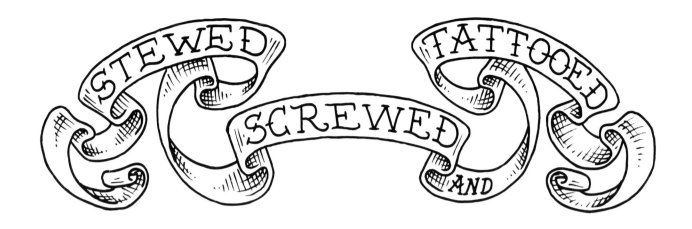

by
Madame Chinchilla

FOR
JEN
Art with a Pulse!
Madame Chinchilla

Archival material supplied
by
C.W. Eldridge
of the Tattoo Archive

Isadore Press
1997
1999

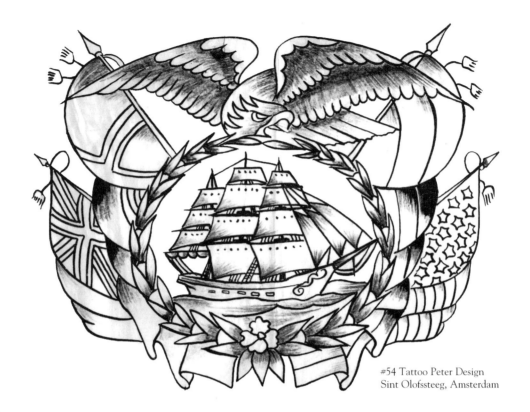

#54 Tattoo Peter Design
Sint Olofssteeg, Amsterdam

Front Cover:
    Madame Chinchilla • Photo: Jan Hinson
Back Cover:
    Captain Don Leslie • Sword-swallower • Tattooed man • Photo: Deirdre Lamb
Publication Layout & Design:
    Chuck Hathaway, Mendocino Graphics, Fort Bragg, California
    Randy Simon and John Dryden, PIXELMEDIA, Mountain View, CA
Photographers:
    Deirdre Lamb Photography • Jan Hinson • Dianne Jasmine • Max Royce
    Triangle Tattoo Museum • Tattoo Archive • Bruno L'Hoste • Chris Wrobleski

Editor: Chris Hart Nibbrig
Proof Reader: June Clark
Editing Assistance: Deborah Grandinetti
PrePress and Production Services: Mendocino Graphics, 155A Cypress Street, Fort Bragg, California 95437
© 1997 Madame Chinchilla
All contents by Madame Chinchilla.

ISADORE PRESS
ATTN: Chinchilla
P.O. Box 1225
Mendocino, California 95460

ISADORE PRESS: Attn: Chinchilla
Triangle Tattoo & Museum
356B North Main Street
Fort Bragg, California 95437

ISADORE PRESS
ISBN 0-9602600-13
Library of Congress Number 94-75673

PRINTED IN U.S.A.

This book is dedicated to my family and to our Foremothers and Forefathers of the World of Tattoo. They have paved our way into this fascinating territory of recording history on the skins of the willing souls who trust us.

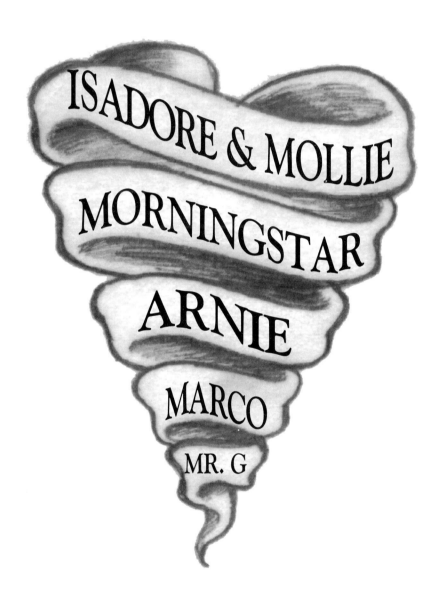

ISADORE & MOLLIE

MORNINGSTAR

ARNIE

MARCO

MR. G

"The authors of the following pages have not only dedicated themselves to the art of tattooing, but also to the soulful endeavors that all of these people undertook in their process of getting tattooed. The stories and pictures are meant to enlighten the social heart and mind. Bravo! To All Living Canvas."

— Max Royce
Photographer

Acknowledgements: Mr. G., Bert Rodriguez, Sailor Mosko David, Lionel Titchener, Captain Don Leslie, Henry Goldfield, Calamity Jane, Crow, Innie Lee, P.A. Stevens, Danny Danzel, Dave Shore, Igor, Lyle Tuttle, Don Ed Hardy, Paul Rogers, Horiyoshi III, Horitoshi I, Krittong Khamlaugwan, Sankom Sakorn, Tong and Chai, Professor Dr. Konrad Spindler, Dr. Hans Moser, National Geographic Magazine, and to all the great tattooers and tattooees.

Thanks to: Daniel Laybourne, Rory Thieman, Jeanne Smith, Jan Hinson, Ron Salisbury, Larry Smith, Ann Sorrel, Lynne Butler and Janice Van Horn, Linda Larsen, Steve Silver, Marco McClean, Cypress House.

Madame Chinchilla's essays have appeared in the following publications: *Mendocino Commentary, Mendocino County Arts Council Newsletter, Mendocino Beacon, New Settler Interview, Sagewoman, National Tattoo Association Newsletter, Tattooing by Women #2-Outlaw Biker Collectors Edition, Tattoo Revue, Borderland, Total Tattoo Book (Warner), and International Tattoo, Tattoo Ink, The Mendocino Outlook, Tattoo International of Oxford, APT, Mendonesian* and *Sonoma County Women's Voices*.

Also by the author: *Longterm Side Effects: Journal of a Woman*, poetry, 1979.

C.W. Eldridge lectures on historical subjects given at National Tattoo Tours and other conventions. He writes for *National Tattoo Association Newsletter; Historian, Archive File, Tattootime, Tattoo Advocate, Native California Newsletter* and *Tattoo World Magazine* by Hanky Panky.

A special thanks to Ron 'Top Dog' Salisbury.

TABLE OF CONTENTS

L I S T   O F   I L L U S T R A T I O N S

Wagner was born in 1875, and had the good fortune of tattooing in New York through the "Golden Age" of tattooing in the U.S. He established himself on the "Bowery", and tattooed there through the Spanish American, World War I, World War II. Charlie Wagner died in 1953. *Courtesy Tattoo Archive*

Percy Waters business card, circa 1920s. His supply business was one of the largest in the world, and his skill at doing large body tattoos was well-known in the show biz world. Waters moved back to his home town in 1938 and lived there till his death in 1952. *Courtesy Tattoo Archive*

Elizabeth Weinzirl card, circa 1970s. Born in 1902, Elizabeth was first tattooed in 1947. Her story was, "My husband wanted a tattooed wife. I wasn't about to move out." So from 1947 up to 1963 Elizabeth got a lot of tattoos mainly from Bert Grimm. Not only was she known as the "World's Number One Tattoo Fan", but at times she was billed as the "Tattooed Grandmother." Elizabeth died in 1993, she will be greatly missed by her adopted tattoo family. *Courtesy Tattoo Archive*

Old Doc Webb business card, circa 1970s. West coast tattooist who spent most of his tattoo career in San Diego, CA. Worked as a commercial artist doing show cards till he met Bob Kelton and began exchanging tattoo designs for tattoo lessons. Bought his first machine from Charlie Wagner in 1926 and spent the next 50 years in the tattoo business. *Courtesy Tattoo Archive*

LIST OF ILLUSTRATIONS

Photo by Deirdre Lamb

removed, clothes were put on the workmen, and tattooing was banished and established tattoo masters found themselves with new customers, the foreigners! The new anti-tattoo law only applied to Japanese, so a tattoo was the ultimate souvenir from this far-off land. This illustration shows a non-Japanese being tattooed in the style of the day, female attendants, food, sake, and music. *Courtesy Tattoo Archive*

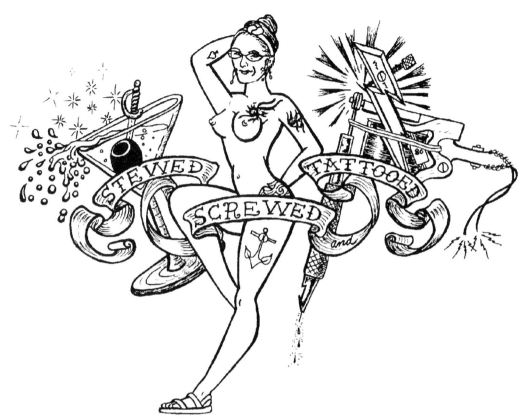

THIS BOOK IS A COLLECTION of stories and photographs of my experiences being a Twentieth Century Tattooed Woman, Artist and Writer, in the fascinating world of tattooing.

The first time I saw tattoos I was five years old. There were numbers on my great, great cousins' arms. My grandmother took me with her when she brought groceries to them. They lived in a dark basement apartment. They were survivors of the Holocaust.

On Saturdays, after Hebrew studies, my father would pick me up, and off we'd go to the Jewish Deli for matzo-ball soup and blintzes. Then I'd go to work with him. I was allowed entrance through back doors with brass plaques engraved "Private" leading to rooms laced with sweet smoke from gooey cigars hanging from the mouths of men looking like greasy dignitaries, their hair slicked back like Elvis.

They wore big diamond rings on their pinkies. Peeking out from their starched white shirt cuffs were markings on their wrists. These were different from my great, great cousins' tattoos.

Being a precocious young girl, I remember reaching over to push up a starched sleeve cuff and seeing pictures that wouldn't wash off: tigers, hearts, naked ladies, dice, four-leaf clovers, and women's names. These became more intriguing than the shiny diamonds or the ornate cigar rings, or even the white powdered-sugar donuts they would give me for being such a good girl, quietly waiting for my father to roll and count quarters from his pinball machines and juke boxes.

Twenty years later, across the street from that smoke-filled room, I got my first tattoo from Zeke Owen in Seattle, and twenty-three years after that I met my mentor and mate, Mr. G. Together we have created Triangle Tattoo & Museum in Northern California. I would never have known then that my first glimpses into the obscure world of tattoos would lead me here.

I want to thank the willing souls who have trusted me to tattoo their precious skins. They have been a pleasure, a challenge and an inspiration for me. None of this would have come to be without the love, skin and support of Mr. G. I feel fortunate to be the controller of my magical wands: my tattoo machines and old silent Corona typewriter.

— *Madame Chinchilla*

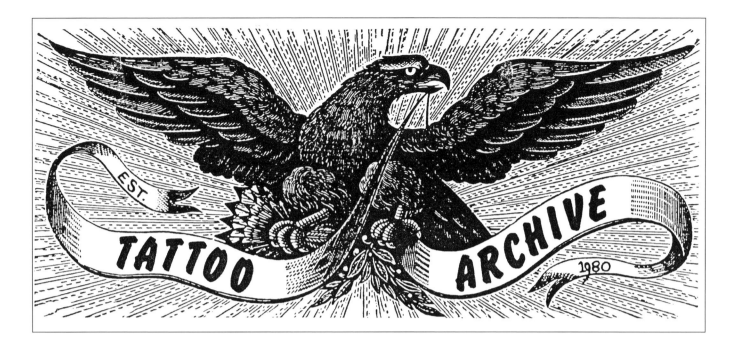

C.W. ELDRIDGE WAS BORN on March 26, 1947, and spent the first 18 years of his life in the Blue Ridge Mountains of North Carolina. He grew up seeing military-related tattoos on many of the men around him and developed an interest in tattoos early on.

Dissatisfied with high school, Eldridge joined the United States Navy in 1965 and set off for a real education. After 13 weeks of boot camp in San Diego, Eldridge was given 12 hours of liberty, about $200 to spend and the first opportunity to fulfill his childhood dream of acquiring tattoos. He returned from liberty with four; the beginning of his personal *scrapbook*. During the mid-1960s, Broadway in San Diego was awash with sailors and all the tattoo shops had lines of white hats waiting for their *marks of manhood*.

After boot camp, Eldridge was stationed in Beeville, Texas, where he often traveled to Corpus Christi to add to his collection of tattoos. In 1967 he was given orders to the aircraft carrier *U.S.S. Oriskany CV 34*, then operating in the Gulf of Tonkin off Vietnam. This ship took him to the Philippines, Hong Kong, Hawaii, and Japan, where he continued to add to his ever-growing tattoo collection. In 1969 he completed his four years of service and headed back to civilian life; spending time at various endeavors including helping organize a rock festival, setting up a bicycle shop, studying welding, and building bicycle frames.

In 1974, Eldridge met and began getting tattooed by Don Ed Hardy. When Hardy decided to open a street shop in the Mission district of San Francisco in 1978, he offered Eldridge a chance to learn the art of tattooing. Eldridge subsequently spent time in Calgary, Alberta, Canada working with Paul Jefferies, in San Francisco with Dean Dennis, and later Henry Goldfield.

In 1980, while working with Goldfield, Eldridge established the Tattoo Archive and in 1984 secured a shop front in Berkeley. A year later, he began working full-time at the Berkeley location. In addition to tattooing, building power packs and traveling tattoo cases for many tattoo professionals, he began actively documenting tattoo history, writing articles for most of the United States and overseas newsletters and publishing *The Archive File*, a quarterly newsletter that is circulated around the world.

In January of 1993, along with Alan Govenar, Don Ed Hardy, and Hank Schiffmacher, he formed a California Nonprofit Corporation named The Paul Rogers Tattoo Research Center after one of the greats in the tattoo business. This organization works toward establishing a national landmark for the art of tattooing.

C.W. Eldridge and his dog Archie live in Berkeley, California, where he spends his free time bicycling and searching for more historical tattoo material.

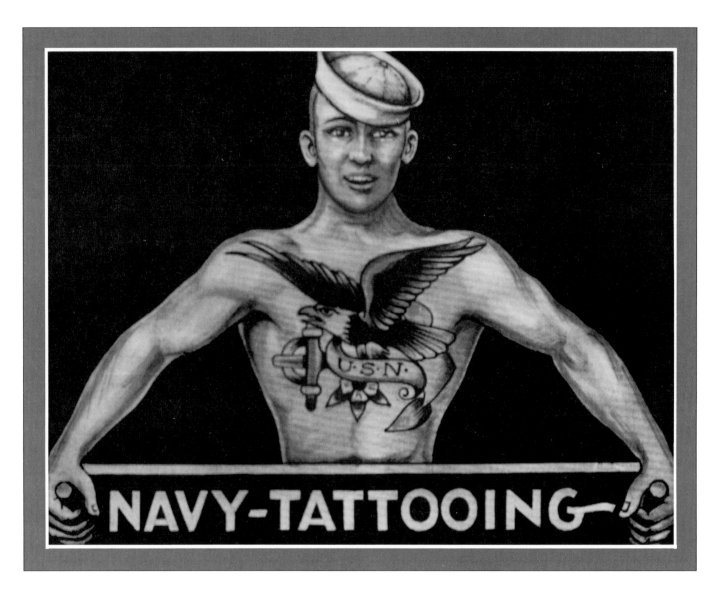

STEWED, SCREWED & TATTOOED

"YEP, I've been all round the world... all over the place. I've even been tattooed by the same tattoo machine as the circus gorilla in 1942. I got tattoos 'cause my dad had 'em. We have a lot of the same ones. My dad is my hero. Hell... I was drunk for most of them. In Sculley Square in Boston, I'd go to the Howard Burlesque... It's torn down now, but we'd go first to the burlesque, and watch all the girly girls wiggle around, then we'd get drunk and rowdy and stagger across the street and all get tattoos.

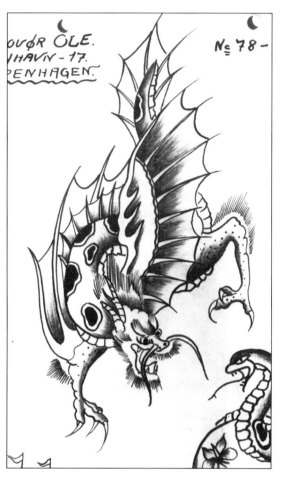

"I was on the Battle Ship USS Arkansas. It was the biggest ship in port. I spent a lot of time on it, and was on my way to Japan when they dropped the Bomb. I was always in the War Zone. I was in Seattle and got the anchor tattoo on my hand, a bunch of us guys got 'em... and we also had sharks tattooed on our other hand. I always wanted Twin Screws... how much are they? I got all these names of my grandchildren tattooed by Lyle Tuttle. I wanted tattoos from the guy... he is famous ya know. When I die, I'm taking my grandchildren with me by having their names tattooed on me. I just love them.

"I'm 68 years old. Ain't I handsome?

"This is my ex-wife's name here on my arm. I've had it for forty years... I'm going to tattoo her husband's name right here... over mine. Yeah... I've been there... done that," he said, as he rolled up his tattered wool plaid sleeve exposing an old time tattoo of a naked lady. "I can even make her dance, wanna see?" We said yes... as he flexed his muscle with vigor and pride. "I got her in '46 in Yokohama. See this bikini... my wife made me put this on her cause she didn't really like the idea of me having a naked lady on my arm, and she made me have her hair tattooed brunette to match hers instead of blonde. That's OK, 'cause I loved my old gal!

"Yep! I've been there done that! Look at this here pig on my foot and rooster on my other one. Got those at Bert Grim's in San Diego... my buddies got 'em too.

"An old seaman's rhyme goes:

Pig on the knee — Safety at Sea
Cock on the right — Can't lose a fight.

"Yep! I'm like an ole leather suitcase now, and I can prove that I've been there and done that.. look at these here names of port on my arm and see these swallows on my chest? I woke up one morning; my head aching and while in the shower noticed my chest hurt and discovered these tattoos. They're just like my daddy's, he had 'em too. Yep! Been there done that... Got Stewed, Screwed and Tattooed but don't remember where that was."

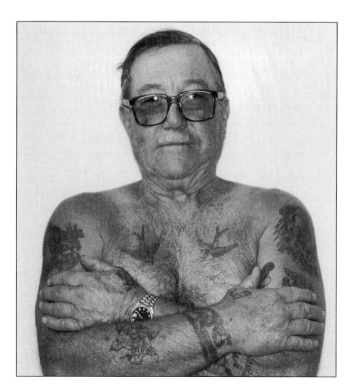

SEAFARING PEOPLE

THE SAILORS FROM Captain Cook's ships, on shore leave in Polynesia, brought tattooing back to England. These sailors were celebrating discoveries and explorations of a dangerous unknown, of vast oceans and new continents. The sailors that charted these new waters were tattooed by natives in seaports worldwide, in celebration of life, discovery, and cross-cultural liaisons. How could anyone at home comprehend their discoveries of paradise and the paradoxes within?

Unfortunately, with time, discovery turned to wars and these men who were about to fight for their country were celebrating possibly the last moments of their lives. In getting a tattoo they were expressing camaraderie, coupled with feelings of fear and loneliness. It was at these times that a lover's name and the word MOM were chosen as a loving symbol to accompany these men on their voyage.

Seafaring tattoos were earned and had significance. When a sailor had sailed 5,000 miles across the sea and back, he had two swallows tattooed on either side of his chest. A tattooed dragon indicated he had crossed the International line, and often a sailor had the name of each port tattooed on the side of his leg. In the British Navy a crucifix tattooed on the sailor's back spared him from a flogging. Sailors in the windjammer days had HOLD FAST tattooed on their knuckles as a safety reminder. Twin screw propellers tattooed on the buttocks served as a talisman for survival if the ship went down. A rooster and pig tattooed on the ankles were to keep the sailor from drowning. Jack London wrote a statement, which I have modernized. It is: "Follow any man [or woman] with a tattoo and you will find a romantic and adventurous past." History has followed these men on leave off of ships, out of saloons, brothels, and into tattoo parlors around the world for centuries. These adventurers were indelibly marking their passages. It may well be that during those 'reckless moments' they were expressing their true form, their innermost self. Ah Yes, 'Reckless Moments'. Life is full of them. In fact, as a war baby, I am one myself.

> *"Every sailor worth his salt had a naked girl tattoo on his thigh, a star and moon on one hand and a small anchor on the other. Then they were considered a top man, fit to drink and fight with the best."*
>
> Doc Webb
> Sailor & Tattooer

LITTLE JIM

LITTLE JIM LIVES IN DOWNTOWN Fort Bragg, California. He was one of the thousands of young men who wandered off their ships in a foreign seaport, and ended up sitting in a straight back wooden chair or lying on a bamboo mat under the incessant buzz of a tattoo machine. He got his first tattoos at the age of sixteen. The tattoos were a black panther and a snake. When he was seventeen, he joined the Navy and was on a 9 CVA 61 Aircraft Carrier. When they docked in Yokohama he wandered into a tattoo parlor to add to his collection of tattoos.

"In Yokohama I got my swallows. One on each side of my chest. I got these because my daddy was a Navy man and he had them too. Swallows are a traditional sailor's tattoo. They signify that a man has crossed the equator and back again. The anchor and chain around my neck were done in San Francisco by Erno at Lyle Tuttle's next to the Bus Depot. The chain has a quick release which is connected to an anchor with a ship's wheel and Jesus Christ is on that; because He carried me through many lives and that is why I carry Him on my back as a sacred tattoo. Although in this life I am a hypocrite, in my last life I was a Viking. My third old lady told me that because I was going to sea all of the time. I still love the sea."

"I suppose, if you could read a person's tattoos you could read his entire life."

— Frank Madera

In times of uncertainty and travel, of war and strife, many men and women got tattoo marks as a sign of permanence in a changing and uncertain world. In the modern world, no matter what the state of the economy, people will always have the means for maintaining and enhancing their self image and for entertainment. The saloons, beauty parlors, bordellos, barber shops and tattoo studios have always had folks trickling through for their necessary selfish pleasures.

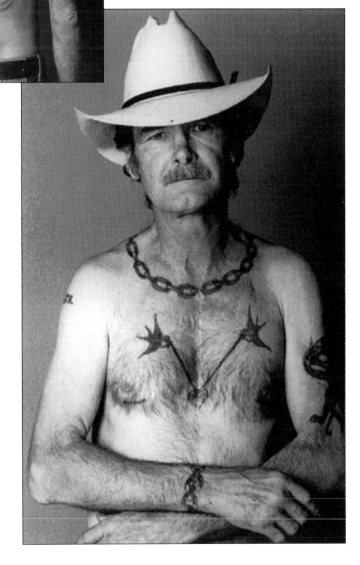

HENRY WAS 17 YEARS OLD and on leave from the Navy when he got his rose tattoo. Shakey Jake (the tattooist), had only one size, it was too big for Henry's arm, so he got it on his chest.

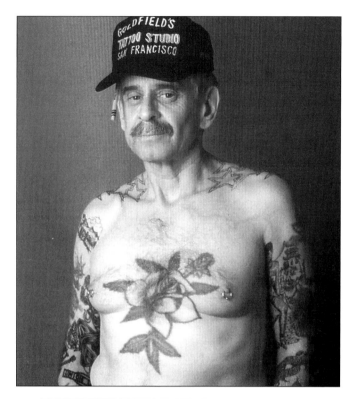

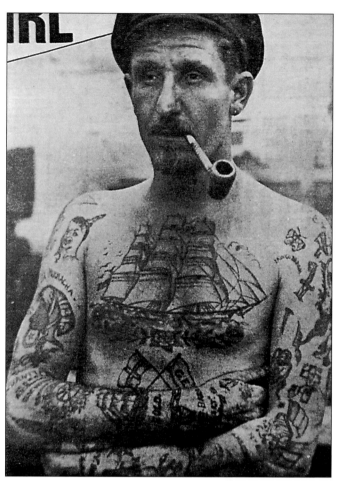

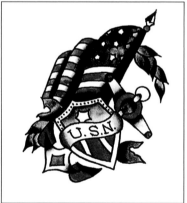

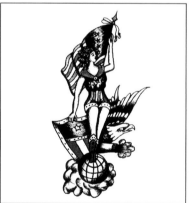

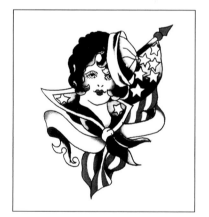

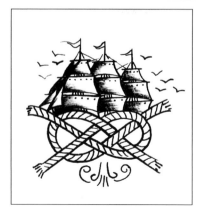

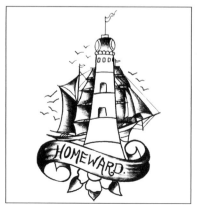

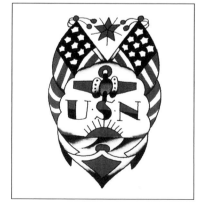

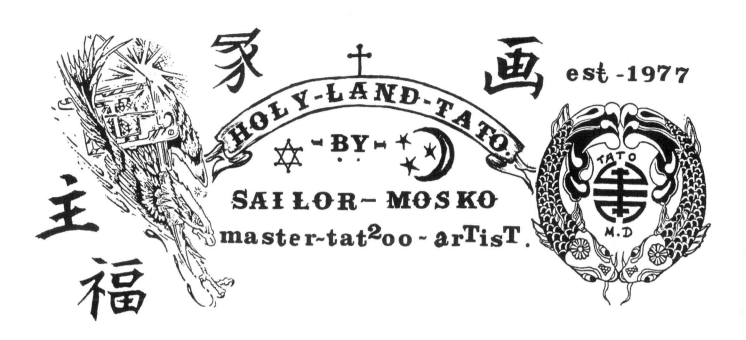

主福 东 画 est-1977

HOLY-LAND-TATO.
~BY~
SAILOR~ MOSKO
master~tat^{2}oo ~ arTisT.

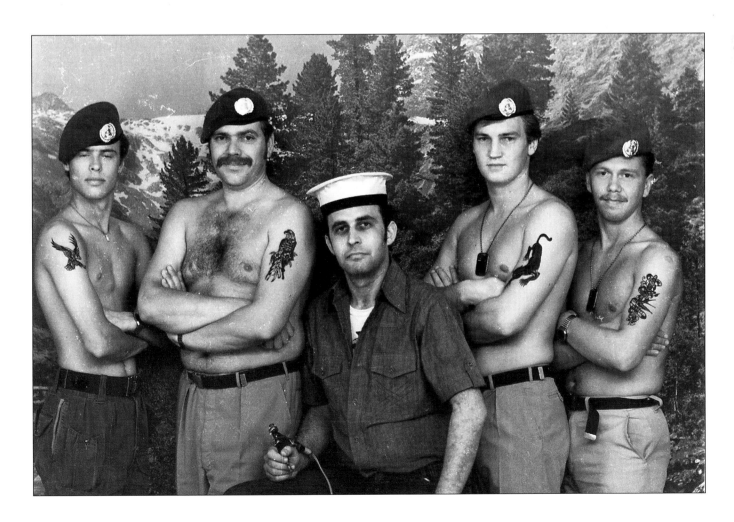

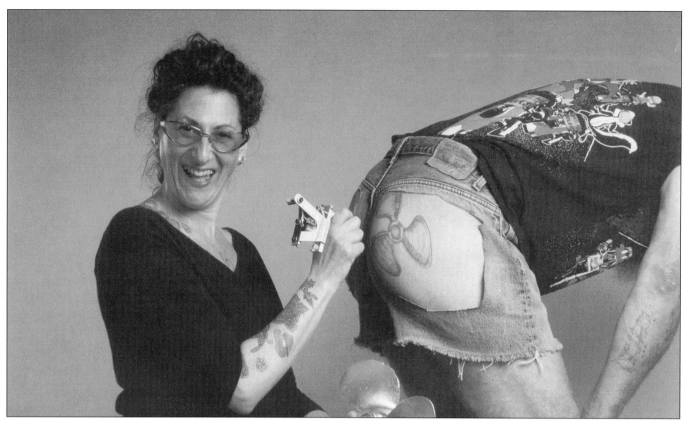

"These twin screw props help propel me through life."
— *Capt. Fuzzy*

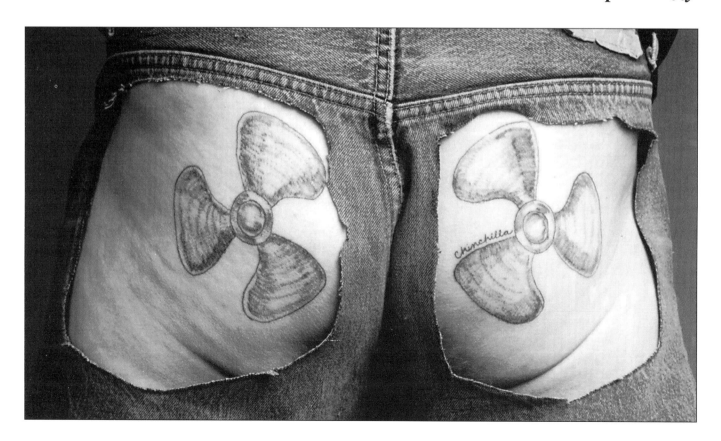

MILITARY

"Coleman used to see his eagles on the chest and laugh his head off. He would put chest eagles on in 12 minutes. He would paint the feathers red, paint the eagle black. He would just do anything to it to hurry it up and give them a little red in the thing. Instead of putting red in back of the eagle he would put it in the eagle wings and wherever."

— Paul Rogers

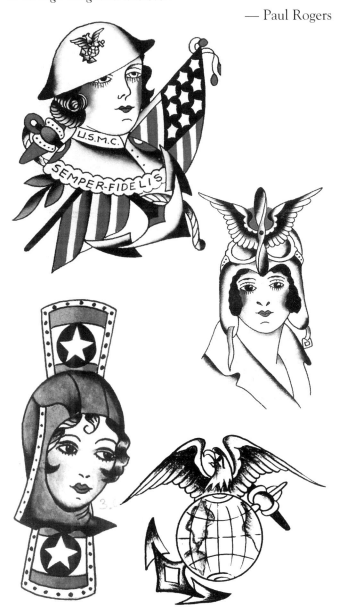

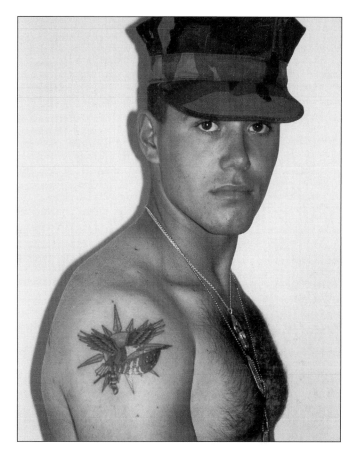

"The reason I got a service tattoo is to represent my service to my county. We don't wear our uniforms, 24 hours a day, but we wear our tattoos for a lifetime. My tattoo is a statement of honor and pride."

"Coleman told the service boys if they were vaccinated he couldn't use green or brown because they would get sick from it. That way he got by just using black and red all the time. It was black and red, black and red, black and red."

— Paul Rogers

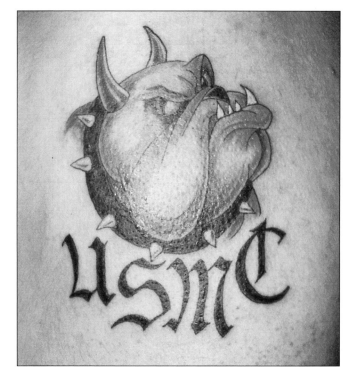

Tattooing has always been associated with warriors. Throughout history many of these warriors did not return home. Some were killed in combat, while others were held prisoner, spending the rest of their lives in captivity. This century was no exception; many American servicemen have been killed on the battlefield, and others have been classified as Prisoners of War or Missing In Action. Robert L. Nessier, Sgt. 1967-1968 Vietnam; pays homage to the MIA/POWs with the POW emblem tattoo on his arm.

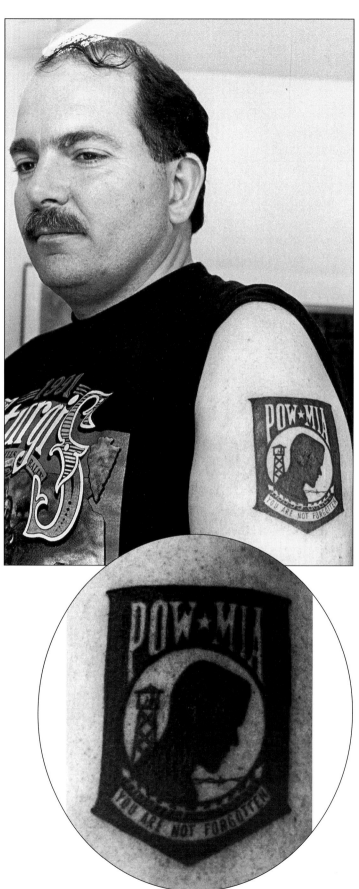

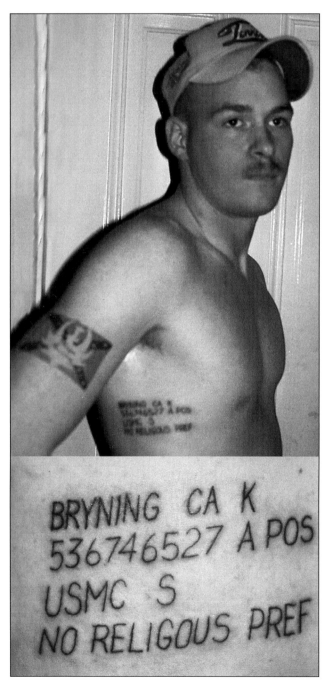

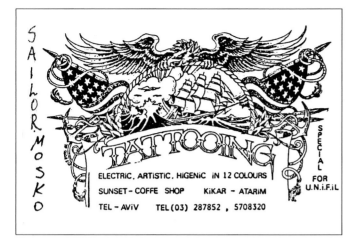

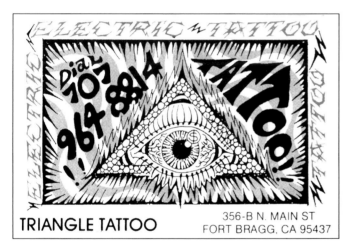

TATTOO BUSINESS CARDS

by C.W. Eldridge

TATTOO BUSINESS CARDS are perhaps the most artistically eclectic; their illustrations encompass aspects of life and death. The art is cross-cultural. One will see everything from butterflies to skulls, as well as slogans and interesting artist's names on them. They are undoubtedly one of the most sought after items of tattoo memorabilia, and a great source of research material for tattoo historians. These cards have vital historical information about the artist and territory of business. Older business cards can be dated by phone exchanges, postal codes and designs.

There is an international list of tattoo business card collectors. To be on their mailing list, contact

Terry Wrigley
23 Chisholm Street
Trongate
Glasgow, Scotland

"Tattoo artist business cards are fascinating bits of history."

— Lyle Tuttle

Tokens of Love

There's tokens, that we treasure,
Some of grief, and some of pleasure;
A lock of hair, a faded flower—
A portrait, or a charm;
But there's one that lingers ever—
And naught but death can sever,
'Tis some loved one's name
Tattooed upon the arm.

Heavy Bright Work   Ladies Work Done
My Specialty   Privately

Prof. Frank Martin

SCIENTIFIC
TATTOO ARTIST
AND
CIRCUS TATTOOED MAN

STUDIO
121 Second Ave., South   (OVER)   SEATTLE, WASH.

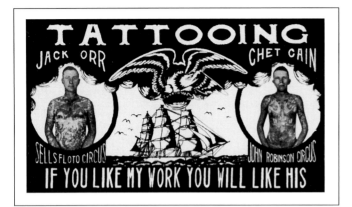

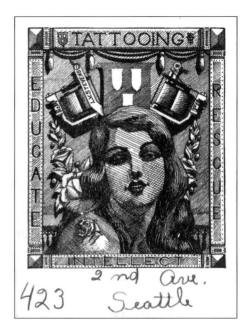

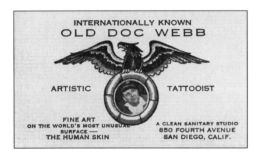

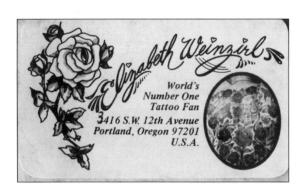

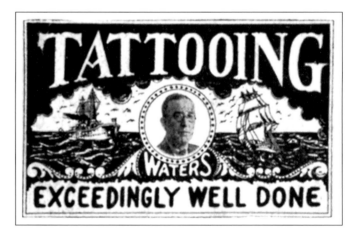

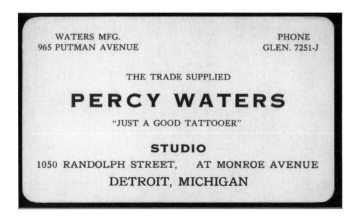

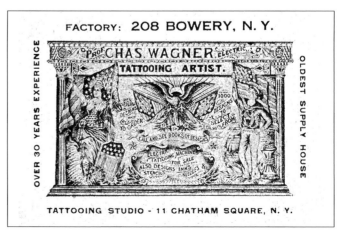

TRADEMARKS

ONE HECTIC SATURDAY AFTERNOON, a man who looked like a cattle rancher walked into our Tattoo studio and asked, "Hey, anyone here wanna see my tattoo?" "Sure," we replied. "Bring me over that there chair." We did, and he sat down and removed his worn cowboy boot, malodorous sock, and exposed his foot revealing a tattoo that had a finger pointing to the big toe which read, "PLACE TAG HERE, Coroner's Use Only." Our visitor was a mortician, saying he and four cohorts decided to get the same tattoo.

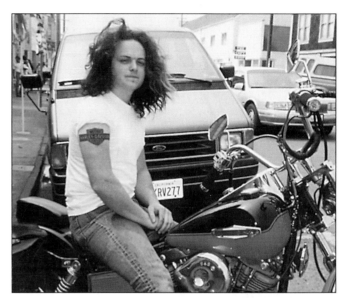

During Redwood Summer, a logger walked into Triangle Tattoo and asked us to tattoo a sawed off red-wood stump on his arm. We did. The following year he returned for a new growth tattooed onto the barren stump. I tattooed a bit of new growth, and he said. "Hell, that's not enough, tattoo more on it." And I did. As he walked out, he turned and said. "See, I'm not such a bad guy after all, the forests do grow back."

A friend of mine from Seattle who owns a nursery came to visit me. Her favorite plant is ivy, so I tattooed a delicate vine winding around her wrist. Other friends in the same business have their favorite flowers tattooed on themselves. Musicians get opening refrains, musical notes, or their instruments as tattoos. The Shakin' Snakes got snakes. We have tattooed the words, NO CODE BLUE on trauma unit caretakers, blood types on jungle doctors, the words BETTER RED THAN DEAD on an Indian Doctor and a full set of wings on the back of a surgeon. A student of Entomology (study of moths), came in for a tattoo of the moth from the movie "Silence of the Lambs."

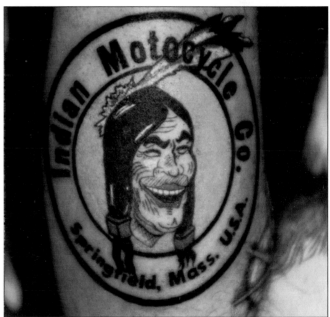

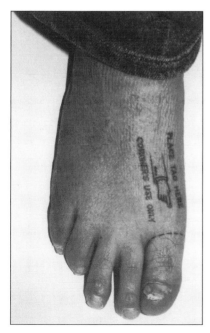

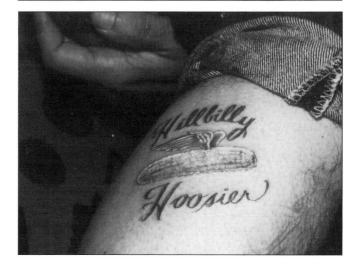

A woman tromped in one windy Saturday afternoon with a plumber's wrench in her hand. She stood there looking around, I told her that she was in the wrong place, our plumbing was working just fine. She laughed, and asked if we could tattoo her wrench with a heart behind it on her back shoulder. And yes, we did.

A husband and wife dressed in matching red striped racing jackets walked in with a photo of a hot red race car, which they wanted tattooed on their arms. It became a sort of an talisman for them. Gamblers and lotto players often have lucky ladies, rabbit's foot, the number seven, dice and four leaf clovers tattooed for good luck. These lucky tattoos have really worked... we won $1800 on the Lotto one year. All Mr. G. had to do was religiously rub each lotto ticket on his lucky lady tattoo for five and a half years!

Artists have miniatures of their paintings tattooed on themselves. A realistic portrait of Elvis surrounded by a cloud of qualudes is alive and well on the back shoulder of an artist who also has a tattoo of a pair of flaming scissors, as she is also a beautician. Another artist, Juanita has a full set of wings on her back that show up only under black light.

A garbage collector got his garbage truck tattooed on his side. A mariner's scene is etched on the back of a professional diver. Max Royce, a photographer has a black and white portrait of her two children tattooed on her back shoulder. Servicemen and women display their colors, pride of country and dedication with tattoos of bulldogs, American flags, eagles, ships, anchors, and abbreviations of their units.

Even we in the tattoo world adorn ourselves with images of instruments of our trade. Some wear their favorite tattoo machine as a tattoo, while others wear Japanese calligraphy that states, "We are Illustrators of the Skin."

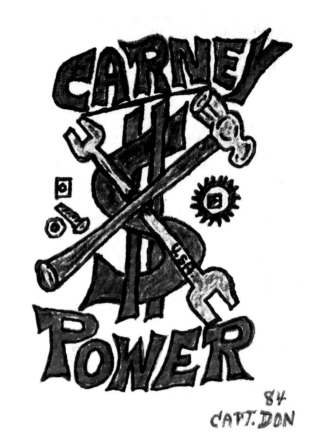

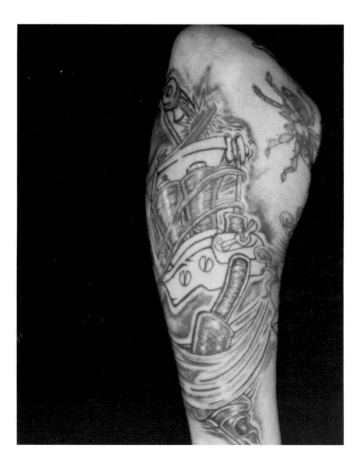

THE MAGIC WAND

by Mr. G.

SURPRISING AS IT MIGHT SOUND, Thomas Edison was the genius responsible for the invention of the electric tattoo machine. In his 1876 patent drawings of a variety of electric engravers lies the blue prints for the tattoo machine we use today. Edison's attempt to modernize the printing industry with it's electric stencil maker forever changed the world of tattoo.

Before the common use and convenience of electric power, tattooing was performed with primitive hand held pokers. These simple and varied instruments

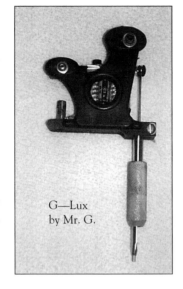

G—Lux
by Mr. G.

"I bought a tattoo kit in 1928. It was a kit from E.J. Miller. He had a supply place in Norfolk, Virginia. The kit ran off dry cell batteries. I did a lot of tattooing on myself back then."

— Paul Rogers

---

remained an unchanged universal method for thousands of years. Whether it was a sharp bone, rock or a ship's sewing needle, basically the hand-poked style was ancient in origin.

It is believed that a tattooist inspired by Edison's invention modified the stencil maker and brought tattooing into the electrical age. As early as 1884, New York's O'Reilly was reported to have a painless electrical tattoo gadget and was the

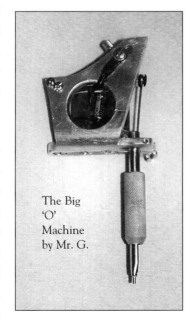

The Big
'O'
Machine
by Mr. G.

sensation on the East Coast. O'Reilly filed for his "Tattoo Machine" patent in 1891. His design was a replica of Edison's rotary contraption, with a flywheel and a new improved two piece tube. O'Reilly had modified an item that was already being manufactured and sold. This machine was soon replaced with another of Edison's improvements on the 1876 drawing. The dual coil reciprocating engraver, a prototype of today's machine, was soon patented by Charlie Wagner.

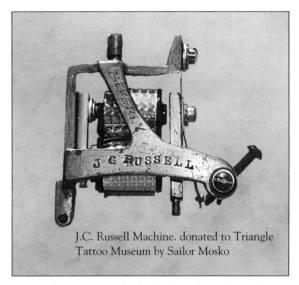

J.C. Russell Machine. donated to Triangle Tattoo Museum by Sailor Mosko

Several tattooists helped develop the electric tattoo machine in to its present form. Percy Waters, Bill Jones, Sutherland Macdonald, George Burchett, Cap Coleman, Jo Kaplan, Micky Sharp, Lionel Titchener, Colonel Todd, Bob Shaw, Lyle Tuttle, Paul Rogers... the list is endless, and everyone has their own way or preference for a brush or a palette.

The tattoo machine is perfectly designed to shade and color, depositing pigment under the third layer of skin. The tattoo machine is nicknamed The Magic Wand by Lyle Tuttle because of its transformational power and function. Lyle Tuttle warmly calls the tattoo machine "Magic Wand because of all the pukes they've turned into Princes."

"Nick Picaro was just a name, this fella Jonesy did all the work. Picaro was a pinochle player. He didn't know anything about tattooing. He used to put a skunk on with green in it or purple or whatever."

— Paul Rogers

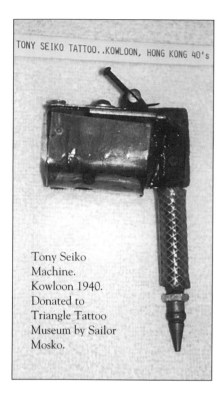

TONY SEIKO TATTOO..KOWLOON, HONG KONG 40's

Tony Seiko
Machine.
Kowloon 1940.
Donated to
Triangle Tattoo
Museum by Sailor
Mosko.

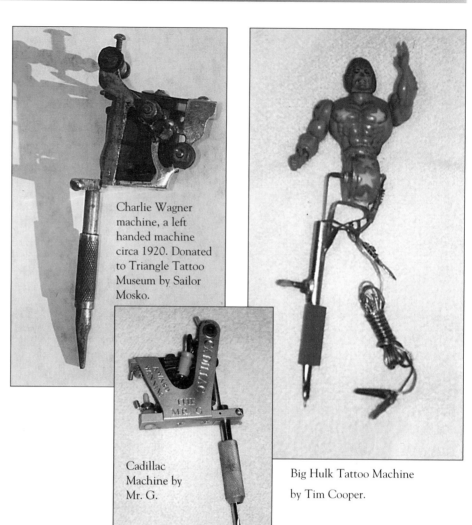

Charlie Wagner
machine, a left
handed machine
circa 1920. Donated
to Triangle Tattoo
Museum by Sailor
Mosko.

Cadillac
Machine by
Mr. G.

Big Hulk Tattoo Machine
by Tim Cooper.

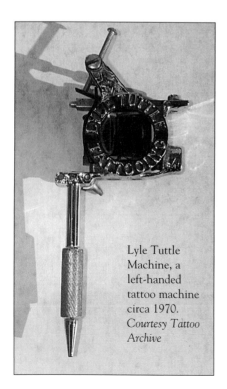

Lyle Tuttle
Machine, a
left-handed
tattoo machine
circa 1970.
*Courtesy Tattoo
Archive*

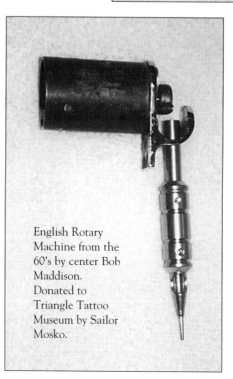

English Rotary
Machine from the
60's by center Bob
Maddison.
Donated to
Triangle Tattoo
Museum by Sailor
Mosko.

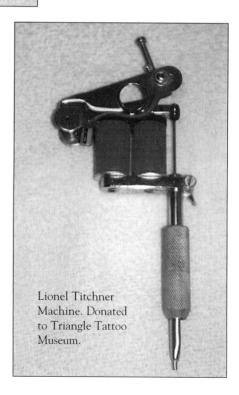

Lionel Titchner
Machine. Donated
to Triangle Tattoo
Museum.

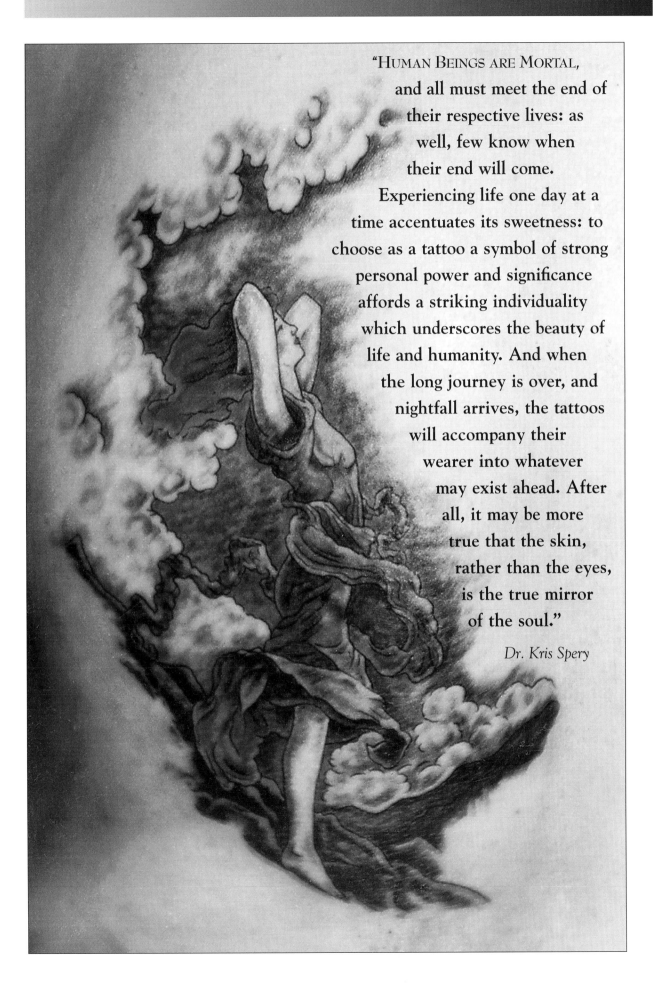

"HUMAN BEINGS ARE MORTAL, and all must meet the end of their respective lives: as well, few know when their end will come. Experiencing life one day at a time accentuates its sweetness: to choose as a tattoo a symbol of strong personal power and significance affords a striking individuality which underscores the beauty of life and humanity. And when the long journey is over, and nightfall arrives, the tattoos will accompany their wearer into whatever may exist ahead. After all, it may be more true that the skin, rather than the eyes, is the true mirror of the soul."

Dr. Kris Spery

SOMETIMES WE GO JUST FOR THE EXPERIENCE

In Honor and Memory of
Asa Lee Crow
August 9, 1941 – November 15, 1996

I'VE NEVER WANTED a spider tattooed on me. I don't even particularly like spiders, but look at me now! It all started with a guy named Asa Lee Crow saying, "Hell, I bet you don't know who I am!"

He was spilling over with stories about his thirty years of gypsy tattooing. We were all ears, and sat rapt as he reminisced, while sitting on our rooftop garden with a slight breeze just barely keeping the fog at bay. Now, a year later, I have his personality captured on video, his face frozen in photographs, and his mark pushed with black ink under the third layer of my skin. A spider. And this is how it came to be.

I asked Crow if I could have a small momento tattoo from him. He said, "Yes, but it will have to be my trademark: a spider."

"A spider!" I replied. "I don't even like spiders."

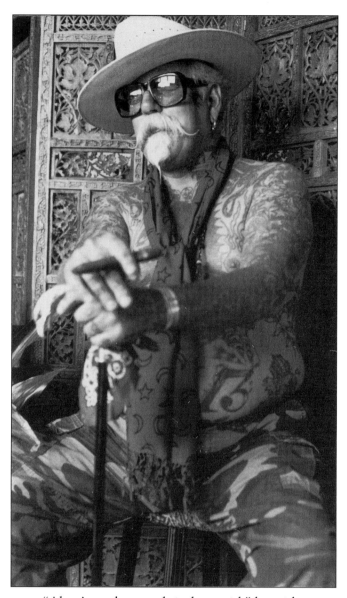

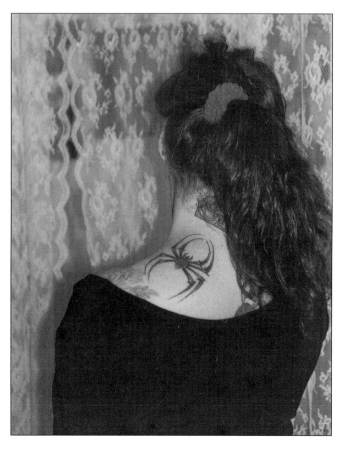

"Ah, c'mon here and sit down girl," he said to me. And like an obedient child I did so, with my dress pushed off my shoulder. Crow drew a spider on my back. I looked at it in the mirror. "Crow, it is way too big. I said a little spider!"

"Ah, c'mon here and sit down and shush up girl," he said to me. And I did so… just for the experience of getting a tattoo from him. Another tattoo story to tell.

When he had completed it, I looked in the mirror. It was elegant, absolutely elegant, and with a smile on my face, I turned to him and sweetly whispered in his ear, "You sure give good spider, Crow."

THE SYMBOLISM OF DEATH IN TATTOOS

THE SYMBOLISM OF DEATH is evident in all cultures. It is expressed through art, poetry, and the rituals of religion. The skull is a commonly used symbol in the world of tattoo art. On my own body, I carry the indelible mark of life meeting death.

I used to have a strong aversion to skulls, because they symbolized death, and death frightened me. But, because of the numerous tattoos of skulls I have tattooed, I view them differently. Now, my aversion is only slight, and I actually enjoy their bare-toothed grimace and rather delight in tattooing a skull, inking its teeth stark bone white. I visited Lyle Tuttle in San Francisco, and bought one of his famous thirteen skull silver bracelets, which I wear as an anklet. At this time of my life, I am wearing fourteen skulls. My back-piece consists of a woman embracing a skeleton. The artist of this piece is Pierre LaComba. Mr. G. did the tattoo. Above their heads is the yin-yang symbol, which represents the balance of life and death. Above are three protective symbols which I received from a Buddhist in Thailand. I chose this tattoo to accompany me throughout my life because of the profound statement it makes about my own mortality. I will eventually surround it with colorful exotic flowers to soften the still disturbing feelings I have about my mortality. The woman in my tattoo is wearing my tattoos. The woman is me, and I am embracing death. I call the piece The Kharmic Embrace.

The image of the skull is not necessarily negative. The skeleton is a symbol of change and rebirth. It is not an image suggesting end in itself but symbolic of another door we pass through. Some people choose a skull for a tattoo in an attempt to defy the fact of their impending demise. But this tattooed statement of defiance is an act of embracing the reality of death. Life is full of doors we pass through, and death perhaps, is the last door to the right.

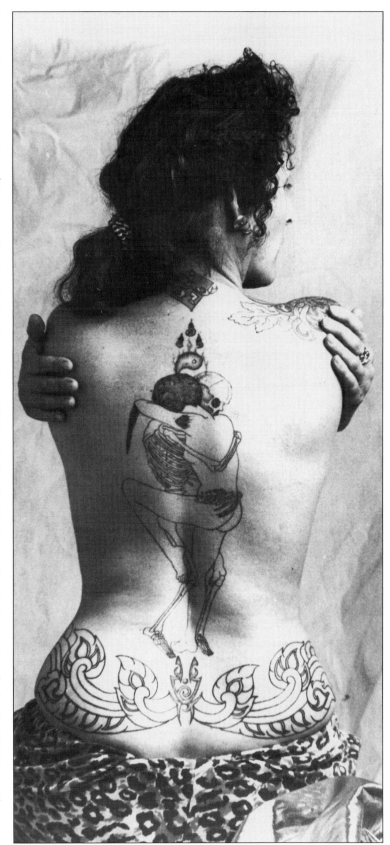

PIGMENTS OF THE IMAGINATION

THE TATTOO ARTIST, image chosen, and the wearer of that image, are conduits linking generation to generation, culture to culture, from the North Pole to the South Pole. The need for ritual is ever present in our society. In the ancient world, tattooing was a ritual that depicted both social and sexual status. It was traditional and decided by the elders. Today the choice is individual. Getting tattooed is a profound act of self-expression. Now we are free to choose the pigments of our imagination, making indelible statements about ourselves and sharing it with the world.

We are the New Tribe, people choosing to indelibly mark our bodies to reflect our beliefs. Perhaps in 2,000 years, we will be exhumed from our respective resting places and categorized as to which tribe we belonged by the evidence of our tattoos. We all know that bad guys are identified by their tattoos. Every time we watch "America's Most Wanted," we see tattoos as part of the description of the convict. In the movies, most criminals have one or more tattoos. In the movie Cape Fear, Robert De Niro was covered with them. Tattooed mavericks are part of the bad scene and traditionally carry with them the socialized images of the "bad guy." Rarely does one see a tattooed "normal" person on the big screen. They are usually anti-social... either outlaws or outcasts.

Thanks to MTV, Cher, Whoopie Goldberg, Roseanne Arnold, The Red Hot Chili Peppers, Vogue, Interview and many other public personalities, the tattoo is staring the public straight in the eye.

Historically, tattooing has been obscure to the general public. It has been a secretive and taboo art practice in the twentieth century. Until recently, the only places to get tattooed have been dark alleyways, back streets and other unsavory locals. Now, as Bob Dylan's song goes; "times, they are a-changing..." Tattoo studios are located on the main streets of towns and cities and are more accessible to the public. Tattoo studios are similar to beauty salons, insofar as they are places where a personal embellishment takes place. Tattoos are personal hieroglyphics, similar to a coat of arms, creating a visual definition of a person's life.

In this century, unlike any other, many profound statements are tattooed on people's bodies.

Requests for tattoos are as individual and diverse as the people desiring them.

"There is a unity of body and mind with the expression of a tattoo. When we ink our skins we choose figures to live with for the rest of our lives. This is not a totem bear on a cord around our neck that we can give away or exchange with revelation. We commit ourselves to mysterious, mythical figures. This is an act of communion."

— Ron Salisbury

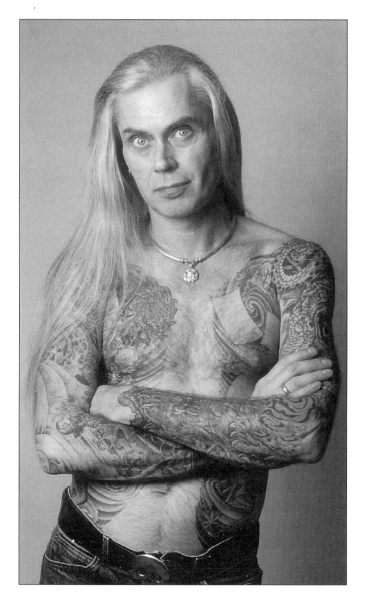

NEW AGE TOTEMS AS AN ATAVISTIC ACT

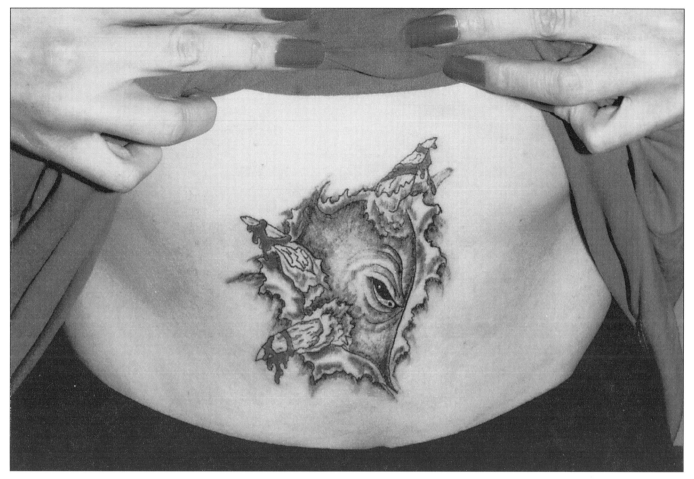

NEW AGE TOTEMS are anything one considers a symbol of personal power; from lucky dice, medicine wheels, crystals, feathers, hearts, and skulls to calligraphy. On my own back I wear a tattooed totem which I call The Kharmic Embrace.

Some totems are carved, sculpted, painted and woven, but ours are pushed under the third layer of our skins. Ancestral memories breathe through our New Age Totems via the ancient Mother Art of Tattooing. We connect ourselves to the ancient world, with these images breathing within our skins. Like a macabre reference library, we are Keepers of the Images. We carry an archive of images and symbols, which have been present worldwide for centuries representing life, death and all that throbs with a vibrant force. These venerated symbols are animal, plant or natural objects and serve as an emblem of a clan or family by virtue of an asserted ancestral relationship.

Mr. G. wears totems which were hand-poked on his back during a religious ceremony by a Buddhist Monk and a Burmese Shaman in the highlands of Northern Thailand. The pigments used were hand-ground red stone, black sumi ink and sacred invisible oils containing herbs, flower petals and amulets. These pigments, unlike ours, are used communally. They are inserted by a sharpened stick of bamboo, brass, or needles made of bone or animal teeth. These sacred tattoos are protective markings, called yantras.

A couple celebrating their first year of sobriety marked their passage with a tattoo of a beast peering out of their belly with a yin-yang eye. They call it the beast within, always remembering their totem.

In a sense tattoos are icons, a tap-root running deeply through cultures for centuries. A lifeline, a point of reference, as well as a form of identification and status, while adorning the body.

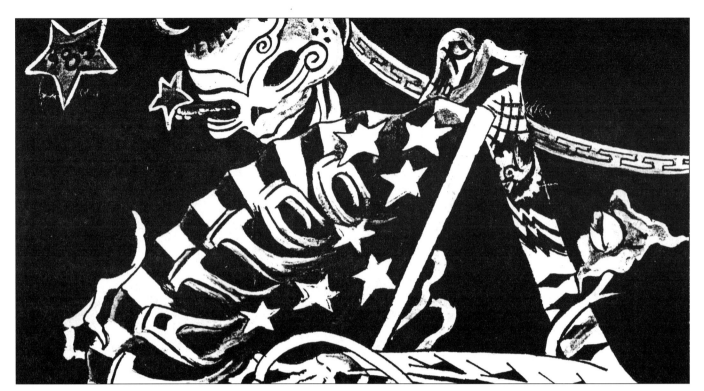

SOCIAL STIGMA & TATTOOS

THE WORD STIGMA ORIGINATES from stigmata, meaning a mark of infamy or disgrace. Throughout European history, tattoos, or other indelible markings, have been considered to be a social stigma. The ancient Greeks indelibly marked their slaves with a delta, while the Romans stamped the foreheads of gladiators who were convicted criminals and sentenced to the arena for easy identification. In the 17th century, Russian courts favored branding and tattooing the faces of criminals. In the early part of the 18th century, the British Army tattooed D for Deserter, and B. C. for Bad Character on the side of the chests of wrong-doing soldiers. This practice was abolished in 1869, and was considered reminiscent of the scarlet letter. In this century, the Nazi regime used indelible markings to isolate the Jews in their prison death camps. In the 1950s, Russian convicts began to tattoo themselves. These tattoos symbolized the hierarchy of prison life, and were considered "Skin-Deep Credentials."

Mythology and religion were also reasons for people to indelibly mark themselves throughout history. The Samoan, Brazilian, Indian, and Mayan cultures all symbolize the "Great Flood" with a line tattooed across the chin. This is a protective mark, saving them from drowning if a flood should occur. Christian and Coptic tattoos are over 400 years old. They originated in Italy. Pilgrims got tattooed as a badge of their pilgrimage across Israel, Spain, and Santiago. It was a three-month trek. A cross tattooed on the inside of the wrist was significant of that crossing. Richard the Lionhearted was one of those crusaders, returning with a cross on his forearm. It was also traditional for the cross to be tattooed on the forehead. In the Coptic region, the cross showed that one was not a Muslim. Emperor Constantine banned facial tattooing.

We are all affected by our socialization. It reaches with a sticky hand into all areas of our lives. It reaches into our work, play, and even our personal image projection. Concerning tattoos; our first were small and discreet, and the initial impact was minimal. But later, with larger, more radical markings, we found ourselves reacting strongly to our new choice of embellishment. There is a point where being tattooed is a profound crossing-over of learned boundaries. It takes strength of character to wear tattoos. The reactions we get are very diverse and interesting. We — the tattooed — are still stigmatized as criminal, insane, dangerous, or just downright individualistic.

Last summer we had a family reunion, during which we posed for the traditional family portrait. Four of us were tattooed. This was the first time my 90-year-old grandmother had seen the large red tribal heart with the curling black flames encircling my delicate arm. She looked at me, then at my tattoo; she touched it and asked, "Is that real?" "Yes," I replied. She gave me that look of love mixed with distaste we are all familiar with and said, "But, darling, you were such a beautiful girl." I smiled and gave her a little kiss on her soft, aged cheek and said, "But, Bobbie, don't you still think I'm beautiful?" "Well yes, darling," she said, "but cover up that arm before dinner."

Mr. G. went to his annual family reunion in the Midwest. It was a humid day when he visited his 90-year-old grandmother. She took one look at him, and pointed to the bathroom saying, "Gregory, you go in there and wash your arms!"

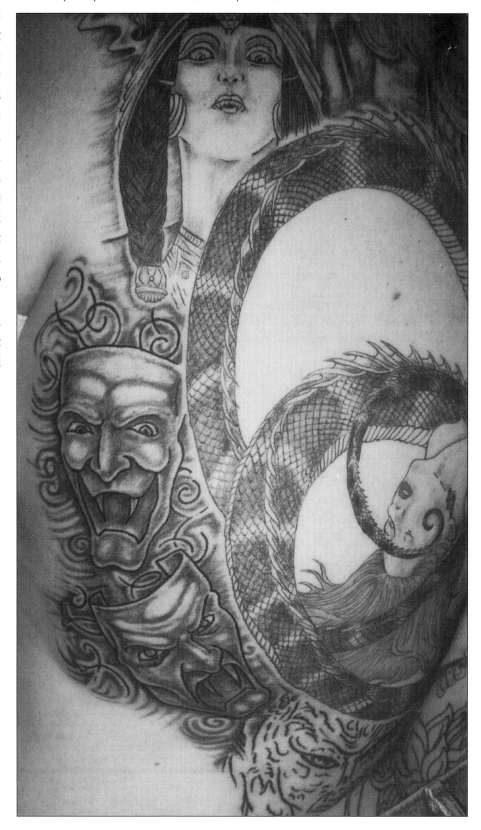

SOCIAL STIGMA AND TATTOOS

TATTOOS ARE EVER PRESENT in my reality. They are extremely fascinating to me, as I am intrigued with their history, the spiritual and psychological aspects of them, as well as the technical and artistic skills involved. And because of this, I have traveled to many countries in quest of this subject.

These are some of the positive and negative responses to being a "tattooed person" in various countries and places of commerce. Our socialization screams out in these few experiences.

Mexico 1991...

It was a typical, hot, stark blue-skied afternoon. We should have been taking a siesta, but instead, we put on sunscreen and sun-hats and ventured for a stroll around the village square. Strolling arm in colorful arm at a coma-like pace around the plaza, smiling lazily and friendly to everyone, we wandered aimlessly for hours. We passed a group of older Mexican women sitting on a bench under a shade tree sipping Coke and smiled at them. A moment later, Mr. G. said, "Did you hear what they called you?"

"No," I replied.

"They called you a 'puta.' 'Puta' means 'whore.'"

I was shocked. It was, as you might think, interesting to say the least. A first for me!

Japan, 1991...

We went to Japan to be tattooed in a traditional hand-poked method by two Tattoo Masters. We stayed in a traditional Ryokin setting with a communal bath, and small rooms with tata-mi mats on the floor for sleeping. In the morning, we walked through the communal area in kimonos and special sandals. The only tattooed people in Japan are the Yakuza, the Japanese equivalent

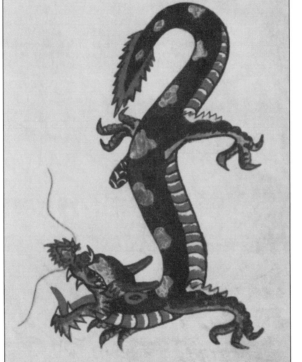

of the Mafia. The Yakuza are not allowed in public baths and are discreet when it comes to exposing their tattooed bodies in public. An elderly Japanese woman caught sight of our tattoos and backed away from us, bowing and saying something over and over again in Japanese, until she was out of sight. God knows what she thought of us!

Thailand, 1991...

We had a few sacred tattoos on our bodies which gained us immediate acceptance and respect with the Thai people. Our other tattoos did not impress them in the least, as they were decorative, not religious in nature.

Supermarket, USA 1992...

One of our tattooed friends was standing in line with his Wonder Bread and a six-pack of beer in Safeway. It was a warm day on the Mendocino Coast, so he was wearing a short sleeved shirt. He was waiting in the 10-items-or-less line, when all of a sudden, he heard a young girl's voice yelling, "Mommy, look Mommy! A Bad Man, like in the movies last night!" Yes, we are being socialized at a young age.

Medical Offices, USA 1992...

A realistic tattoo of a heart is emblazoned on the chest of local artist and salsa disc jockey. He is particular to whom he will open his shirt and share his heart. He went for his physical examination, and when the doctor went to listen to his heart with the stethoscope, he was aware of Eduardo's tattoo. He invited the medical staff in for a look at the two-hearted man.

Acupuncturist, 1992...

Zvika, a new local acupuncturist, gave Mr. G. and me treatments for our common ailments of aging, aching, etc.... It was an artistic as well as a healing experience for us, as the needles pierced the tiger on Mr. G.'s arm dead center in the eyeball. The Chinese God,

Nezha, on the back of my neck was punctured in his little head. We have micro photos of this.

Last week, I tattooed an Indian Rainbird ankle-band on my brother, and Zvika applied acupuncture needles as an anesthetic. It was partially effective and unnerving at the same time!

Physical Therapy, 1992…

My physical therapist asked me if we knew a guy with a back piece of Jesus crucified on an anchor. She said she had never given Jesus ultra-sound before, and how surreal the experience had been!

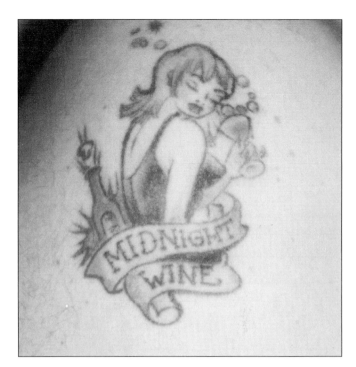

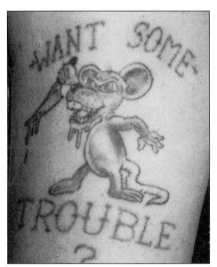

As tattooed individuals, we use our bodies as an artistic medium of expression. We change what we have the power to change. We feel somewhat powerless when it comes to changing the world, but empower ourselves with our decision to embellish our bodies.

Art has always mirrored the zeitgeist of the times, tattooing included. It is a primitive act, and an ancient practice in this technological age.

Needless to say… being a tattooed person can be challenging.

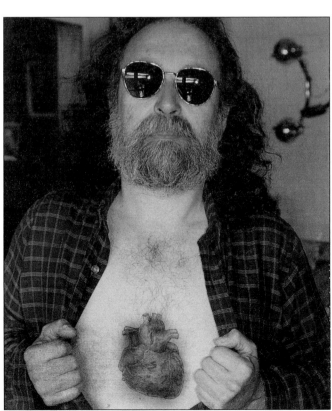

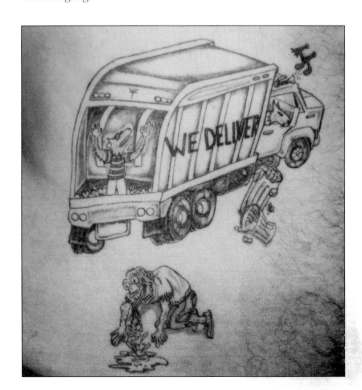

SOCIAL RESPONSIBILITY AND TATTOOING

"TO MARK SOMEONE FOR LIFE is a great responsibility that involves a deep understanding of the history and craft of tattooing. This is passed down to us by our teachers, some of whom have passed on, some are from Japan, Burma, and the United States. Whoever marks a person is responsible for all whom he marks. This process is deeper than we wish to acknowledge. The tattoo artist initiates the ceremonial process with the person who wants the tattoo. And even though there are no drums beating or chanting, this is perhaps the oldest ritual on earth." — Mr. G.

Youngsters come up to Triangle Tattoo & Museum and linger boggle-eyed, at the many designs on our walls. We often engage them in conversation, asking which tattoo they would want if they were eighteen. The boys predictably point to the grim reapers, bulging-eyed skulls, and fierce tigers ripping out of bloodied skin. These are their choices, and thank goodness for the invention of the removable tattoo, so these youngsters can live out their fantasies in a transitory way. The young girls usually want a pretty flower, unicorn or butterfly. It is interesting they are not radical in their choices, but more peaceful and typically less violent.

A young man in the midst of his angry stage of life walked up our stairs requesting a tattoo of the word "EVIL" in Japanese calligraphy. I asked him why, and he replied, "There is a lot of evil in the world. That's why I want the tattoo." I told him that I could not tattoo that on him or anyone, and that a vibration accompanies each tattoo. But I would tattoo it backwards, which spells "LIVE." He agreed. His mother called to thank us for our decision and now he also thanks us, and feels that it changed the energy in his life in a positive manner.

There are certain tattoos that we refuse to do. They include any racist or gang-related symbols, or anything that has a negative or angry slogan or meaning. Only on particular people will we tattoo the words FUCK YOU, and this is most commonly done on the inside of the lower lip.

We feel responsible for what we tattoo on a person,

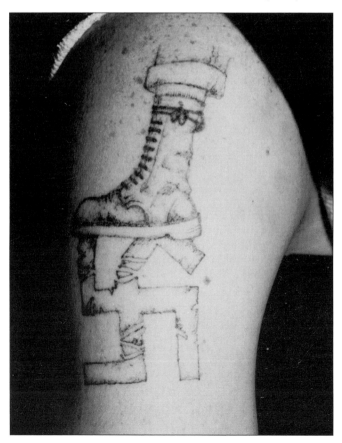

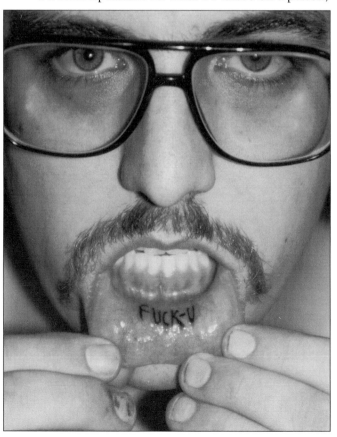

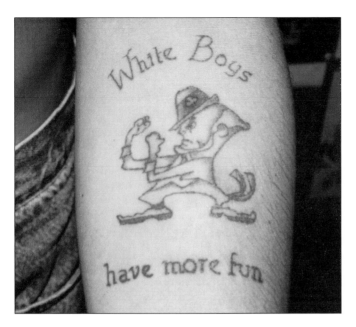

as it is an indelible statement, and wherever the person goes the statement goes with them.

We will not tattoo hands or faces, as we do not want to assist a person in hindering their interaction with the world. We don't want the responsibility.

Names are another touchy request. I will tattoo names on women if they insist, but only in a pastel color. The reason being that pastels are easier to cover up if necessary, than a black-lettered name. Many women have thanked us for doing so, after the loves of their lives changed.

A woman came in for the tattoo of a ribbon around the name of her husband of twenty years. His name was

Hank. She said, "Leave a little room on each side of the name in case we break up. Then, I will come back for the letter 'T' in front of Hank, and the letter 'S' on the end, spelling "THANKS." That was a woman thinking ahead!

Being a mother and woman, I have a different sensibility than some male artists, and react differently to tattoo requests. For example, if a young man wants a tattoo on his forearm, unless he is already tattooed there, I will suggest putting it on his bicep, as I feel it's wise for them to have the option of wearing a shirt sleeve over their tattoo when looking for work. The social stigma of wearing tattoos is lessening, but still prevalent and can affect an employer's decision to hire someone or not.

Most people want tattoos that express their identification with certain images. It is interesting to hear individual requests. I am often shocked. Once, a seemingly conservative hairdresser came in for a tattoo of a butterfly on her neck. I told her that she was "outdoing me" in being so radical in her request, and was she sure she wanted it there? "Yes," she replied, and now she has this wonderfully colorful butterfly sitting on her graceful neck in full view of the world around her. Her husband, who is a school teacher came in for a matching one. I am often amazed at a person's request for tattoos, and even now, as I catch a glimpse of my own tattoos in the mirror, I feel curiously amazed.

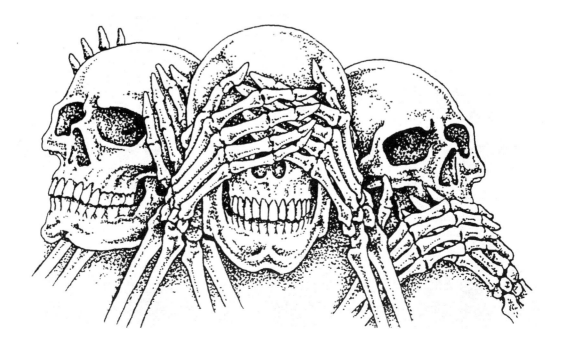

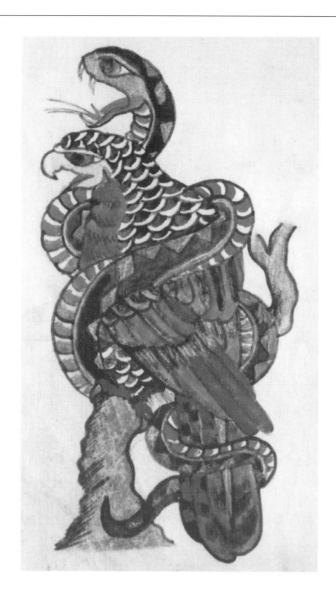

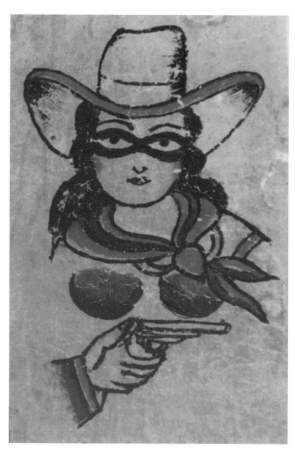

ANCIENT RITUALS

TATTOO STUDIOS ARE IMAGE ARCHIVES. These images represent all areas of life and death, fantasy and reality. They encompass all emotions. The walls are so laden with literally thousands of mythic, fanciful and artistic images, you may feel over-stimulated, confused or assaulted by the energy of them. In front of you may be a torn and bleeding eyeball, hanging by a sinewy thread from a skeleton's eye socket, his bone-white hand reaching pleadingly toward you, or a bat flying in the misty background in the blue eerie light of the waning moon. And next to it may be a display of colorful butterflies drifting through pastel smoke or amongst delicate flowers. To your left may be dense black new tribalistic designs. And from one of these many patterns you may hear one boldly speak to you, saying, "Yes, choose me, I will look great wrapped around your arm or leg or perhaps flowing across your muscular or delicate shoulder."

When you see the design that is right for you, it will speak to you. We have been spoken to many, many times.

DRIED DRAGON'S BLOOD AND MUMMY DUST

IMAGES HAVE BEEN TATTOOED into the flesh for centuries. The process is always the same, an abrasion of the skin and the insertion of pigments that are, in most instances, permanent. The materials used are made from different concoctions, and most of them are secret recipes, similar to a witches brew or the mysterious elixir of the gods.

Ole Phil Sparrow, a tattoo artist from Chicago and Oakland in the '50's, said that he put Dried Dragon's Blood and Mummy Dust into the tattoo inks to make folks come back for more tattoos. We tell our customers that we put Come Back in our inks.

Sankon Sakom, the powerful Monk in Chaing Mai, Thailand, pushes invisible sacred oil, ground red stone dust or black pigment under the skin while chanting prayers in a ritualistic manner.

Krittong, the Shaman who tattooed us in a remote village in North Thailand, used his own concoction of sacred oil, amulets, plant leaves, and flower petals, mixed with black pigment. This was used only in conjunction with chanting and prayers, and for healing and magical purposes.

Horitoshi I and Horiyoshi III of Japan used Sumi ink, which is made by chanting monks, hand ground and mixed with a liquid which creates a very dense black pigment.

In India the women mix ash with kerosene to tattoo themselves. Their line and dot patterns heal a bluish-black, which is a tantric symbol for energy and power.

Thorns, fish bones, sharp pieces of obsidian and various bones have been used to penetrate the flesh in order to insert the pigments.

In prison, the soot from burning bibles, cellophane and such have been used as pigment for tattooing. Shoe polish mixed with saliva is used.

The pigments are elixir in a sense. Their purpose is to make and leave an indelible mark on the flesh and the symbols and meaning are as varied as the colors of the spectrum.

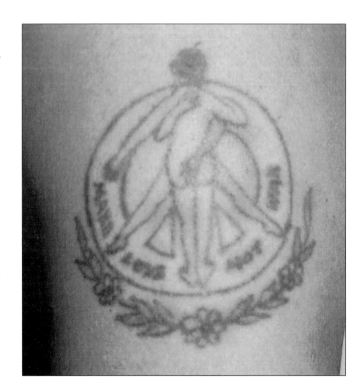

WARNING:
TATTOOS MAY BE ADDICTIVE

LUCKY LADY WINS LOTTO

LUCKY LADY TATTOOS ARE USUALLY naked ladies surrounded by dice, rabbit's feet, four-leaf clovers and are sometimes found sitting haphazardly in an over filled martini glass. They are worn like talismans.

Mr. G. wears one on his dice-throwing arm. She is a design from an old Sailor Jerry Design, popular in the 40's. She has red hair and straddles an obscure tattoo machine with a four-leaf clover tattooed on her bum. Surrounding her are dice and a rabbit's foot. Crowning her head are four playing cards, all the ace of diamonds.

Every Wednesday and Friday we buy Lotto tickets, using our lucky numbers and quick picks. Directly after purchasing them, we rub them vigorously on Mr. G.'s Lucky Lady tattoo, I kiss them, and then they go into his wallet till 8:30 when we call for the results, or we wait till the Sunday rag comes out. We have been religiously doing so for five years, and alas! One rainy evening we sat cozily next to our warm wood stove, the rain and wind howling outside the door. Mr. G. said, as he says every Wednesday and Saturday nights. "We might be millionaires." It happened to be a Sunday evening we had been gone all day and were just settling down for the night with a hot cup of tea and the Sunday paper, when he said, "Oh, shit… Oh, shit… Oh, shit… Oh, shit… Oh, shit!" I asked "Oh, shit what?" He read the numbers off to me. We got five outta six numbers that dark rainy night-$1800 big ones!

Mr. G.'s Lucky Lady tattoo paid off, so now we are trying for six numbers!

[*This money bought our tickets to Thailand.*]

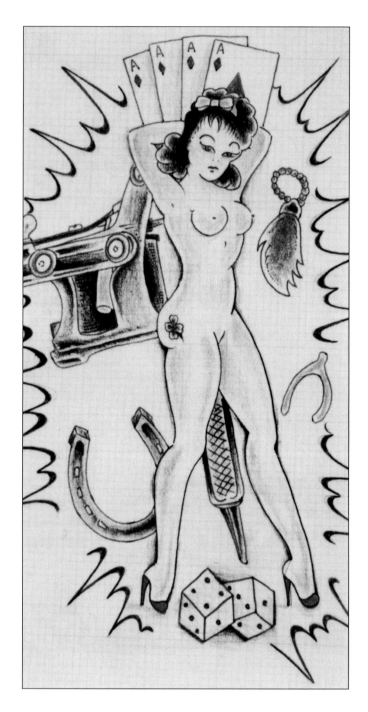

EACH TATTOO IS A CATHARTIC EXPERIENCE

SWIRLING IN THE DREAMLIKE substance of our DNA are ancient images. Atavism rises like the phoenix out of the flames onto the surface of our skins.

We give life to these images that lay await in the dreams of sleeping creatures, in the shadows of history, on the walls of caves and tattoo studios, and even between the musty pages of ancient books.

Rising out of the cauldron, these images will agonize feeling the first sting of their birthing, their first gasp of fresh air, and the first glimpse of the blinding light. Their emergence will create an exultation impossible to describe.

Breathing in a quiet fury, these images will pulse beneath our skins. We have released them from the ether, the nether world.

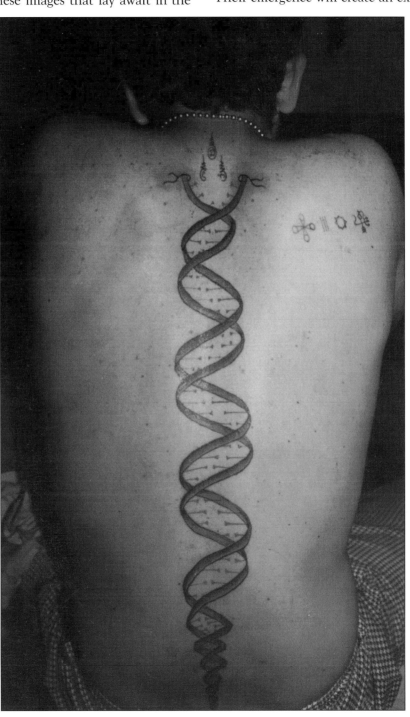

at•a•vism (át´_-víz´_m)—n. 1. The reappearance of a characteristic in an organism after several generations of absence, caused by a recessive gene or complementary genes. 2. An individual or part displaying atavism. [Fr. atavisme <Lat. atavus, ancestor : atta, father + avus, grandfather.] at´a•vist n. at´a•vis´tic adj. at´a•vis´ti•cal•ly adv. [1]

1. *The American Heritage Dictionary*, (Houghton Mifflin, 1987), Microsoft Bookshelf 1992, s. v. "at•a•vism."

MADAME CHINCHILLA

MANY OF YOU READERS out there might be curious or thinking to yourselves: "What's with this MADAME CHINCHILLA tattoo across her shoulders? Is it real? Why would anyone in their right mind want to get their own name tattooed on themselves? Is she forgetful? Or did she have it done because no-one else will have her name tattooed on them?"

There is rhyme and reason to this tattoo. As I was researching circus tattooing for our Circus Sideshow Attraction Exhibit, Chuck Eldridge, the Tattoo Archivist, informed me that tattooed sideshow attractions often had their name tattooed across their back, chest, or stomach for identification.

I was showing tattoo artist Les Pain an illustration of Belle Irene; a tattooed circus sideshow attraction, and one of Captain Don Leslie; sword-swallower, fire-eater, and tattooed attraction; both sporting their own names on their tattooed bodies. Les said to me, "Let's do it." I asked, "Let's do what?" He said, "Let's tattoo MADAME CHINCHILLA across your shoulders, you have room for it, look… right here." He pointed to the wide expanse of virgin flesh on my back, and as I looked over my shoulder in the mirror…without a second thought I replied… "OK, Why not?"

The next day we decided to do the tattoo. I found an alphabet which was a mix of old English and Art Nouveau, and customized it. Then we laid the design on my back and after three hours of being the receiver of the incessant stinging buzz of the tattoo needles, I am now easily distinguished from any other tattooed person in the world. And if I become lost and have amnesia, all one has to do is look on my back and identify me.

Also, perhaps when I am older, I may have Alzheimer's and end up in a nursing home. If so, I can envision myself shuffling down the hospital corridor, gripping my walker with bony hands, my hospital gown open in the back… I can just see myself with a lost look on my face and asking… "Who am I? Who are you? Where am I?" and feeling a gentle hand on my shoulder, hearing the volunteer tell me… "You are Madame Chinchilla, your name is tattooed on your back, look

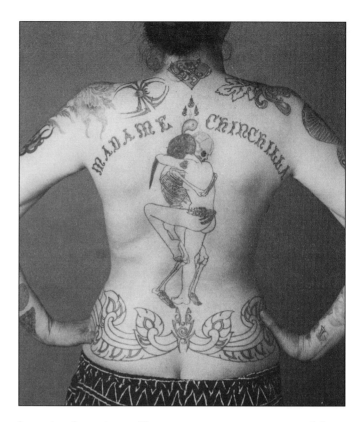

here in the mirror. You were a tattoo artist on Main Street in Fort Bragg, California at Triangle Tattoo and Museum forty years ago. Look at your tattoos… Do you remember?" And I imagine gazing at my image in the mirror and feeling horrified, grasping my chest and dropping dead at the sight of myself!

I was going to donate my organs to science, but after learning that they would just float in a plastic bucket full of formaldehyde, I decided against it. Then I was going to donate my skin to the Tokyo Skin Museum, in fact, it is in my will, but I doubt if it will be terribly interesting for them, as I only have two Japanese tattoos and am mostly wearing tattoo Americana-style designs; so I decided to also state in my will that I want to be heavily embalmed and put in a simple wooden box. On the bottom of the box I want a small two-inch high by one-inch wide door cut and hinged onto it. Then the door will be ornately decorated with a small sign: ART MUSEUM. After my casket is lowered and before they cover it with dirt, I insist the door is left ajar for my many little forthcoming visitors.

NOTE: *This column was inspired by Circus Sideshow Attractions and the death of a family member.*

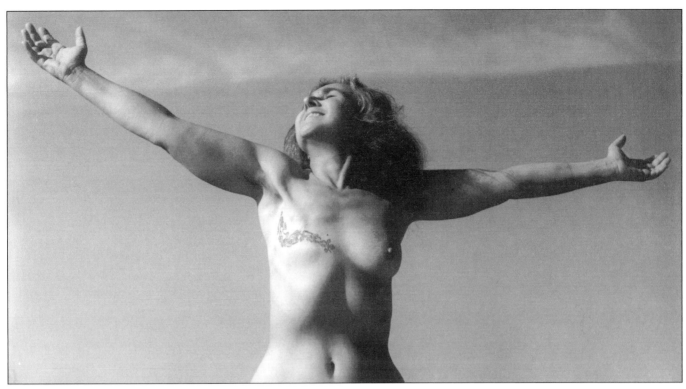

Photo of Deena Metzger • Photo by Hella Hammid

IN CELEBRATION OF A SCAR • SUNDAY, AUGUST 1, 1977

"I am no longer afraid of mirrors where I see the sign of the amazon, the one who shoots arrows. There is a fine red line across my chest where a knife entered, but now a branch winds above the scar and travels from arm to heart. Green leaves cover the branch, grapes hang there and a bird appears. What grows in me now is vital and does not cause me harm. I think the bird is singing. When he finished his work, the tattooist drank a glass of wine with me. I have relinquished some of the scars. I have designed my chest with the care given to an illuminated manuscript. I am no longer ashamed to make love. In the night, a hand caressed my chest and once again I came to life. Love is a battle I can win. I have the body of a warrior who does not kill or wound. On the book of my body, I have permanently inscribed a tree."

— Tree

This is an excerpt from her book Tree, *available from:*
P.O. Box 186
Topanga, CA 90290

Tattoos, wrinkles and scars are external marks of our life experience. The feelings which accompany them vary from a sense of pride to a feeling of aversion. Transformation through tattooing over a scar can have a powerful effect.

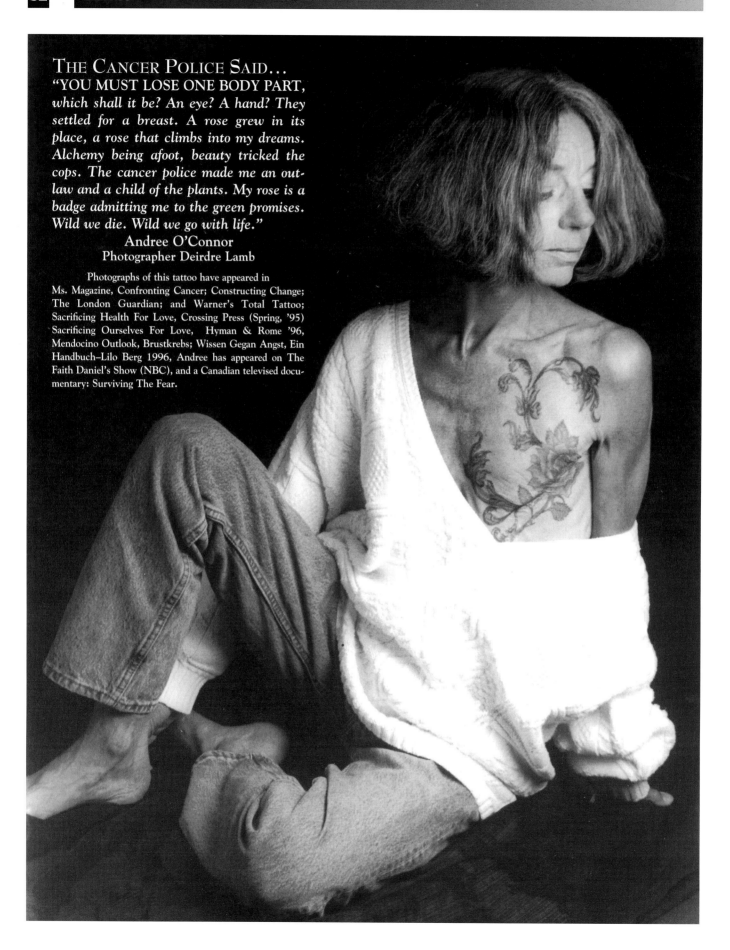

THE CANCER POLICE SAID...
"YOU MUST LOSE ONE BODY PART, *which shall it be? An eye? A hand? They settled for a breast. A rose grew in its place, a rose that climbs into my dreams. Alchemy being afoot, beauty tricked the cops. The cancer police made me an outlaw and a child of the plants. My rose is a badge admitting me to the green promises. Wild we die. Wild we go with life."*
Andree O'Connor
Photographer Deirdre Lamb

Photographs of this tattoo have appeared in Ms. Magazine, Confronting Cancer; Constructing Change; The London Guardian; and Warner's Total Tattoo; Sacrificing Health For Love, Crossing Press (Spring, '95) Sacrificing Ourselves For Love, Hyman & Rome '96, Mendocino Outlook, Brustkrebs; Wissen Gegan Angst, Ein Handbuch–Lilo Berg 1996, Andree has appeared on The Faith Daniel's Show (NBC), and a Canadian televised documentary: Surviving The Fear.

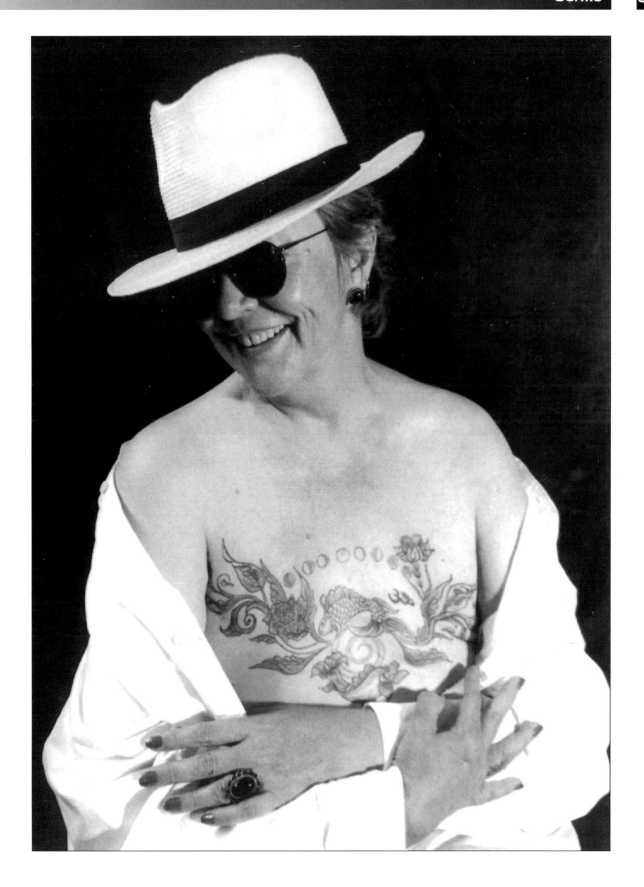

"Shoot The Dice – Have Your Fun!"

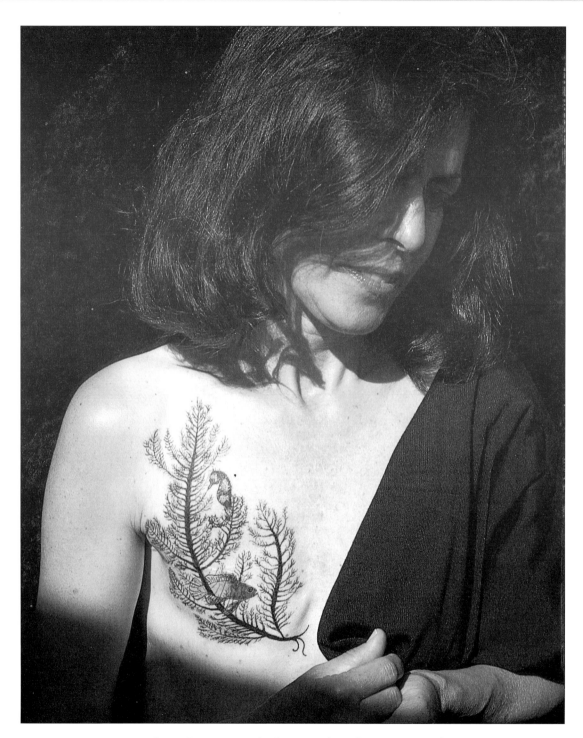

I HAD ALWAYS FOUND PLEASURE and comfort in my naked visits with myself in front of my mirror. My mastectomy robbed me of that private joy. Four years passed and my sorrow grew and finally got my attention.

The a dear friend of mine showed me a photograph of a woman who had this lovely rose tattooed on her body where one of her breasts had been. She looked lovely. I was impressed and excited, but also afraid.

With my friend's loving persistence, I chose a design that was meaningful and very dear to me. Then I mus-tered up the courage and in two sessions, I accomplished more than I had ever hoped.

I cannot explain why or how this tattoo on my chest made it possible for me to feel whole again. But it has.

Now when I stand in front of my mirror, the woman I see and love is happy and eager again. I am grateful to have her back.

Linda Marie

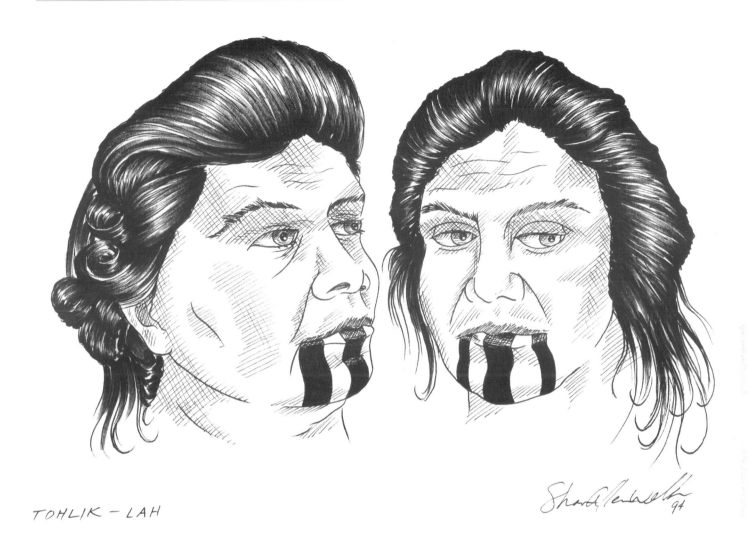

TOHLIK — LAH

On February 9, 1990 the Tattoo Archive was honored when two native American women, Beverly Nix Walsh and Bertha Peters Mitchell came to our studio to have their traditional chin tattoo done. Generally this tattoo would have been done when these women were quite young but because of family pressures they waited until later in life. These women are from the Pohliklah tribe of Northern California, (sometimes called Yurok) and it had been over 100 years since any women in that tribe had been tattooed with the hundred-and-eleven, as their tattoo marks are generally called. This was not a spur of the moment decision for these women, they said they had thought about having this done for over ten years. All of the native people who could have done this tattooing had died off. A local writer mentioned the Archive to these women and as they say, the rest is history. It was a technically challenging tattoo since stripes had to go all the way into the mouth, certainly an area I had never tattooed before! It was a spiritual challenge as well and has altered my idea of what tattoos are about.

— *Sherry Markwart*

TATTOOING AMONGST THE TRIBES OF CALIFORNIA

WITH THE DISCOVERY of fire emerged the primitive urge for men and women to mark themselves in distinguishing manners. Tattooing is a significant enduring art form in the Tribe of Man. It discerns the Warrior, the Goddess, the Medicine Man, the Virgin, etc. It is a ritual similar in spirit to baptism, circumcision and scarification, transforming one's physical image, as well as the sense of self, and even deeper, one's psyche. It links us to one another from generation to generation… from North Pole to South Pole.

Tattooing was prevalent among most California tribes. Both men and women were tattooed, but with different designs signifying status, cultural roles, religious and tribal identification. The tattooing was done in a ritual manner by a designated member of the tribe whose primary function was to tattoo and pray. The person was called a medicine man or shaman.

One instance of pre-pubescent tattooing was among the Tolowa. It was believed to help them in their growing process. Facial tattoos were seen among the Sacramento Valley women, they consisted of dots, zigzags and lines. Only on the Mendocino Coast were the Indians tattooed on their nose, with designs of dots and circles. Facial tattoos were purely aesthetic. Vertical bands were tattooed on the chins of many tribes, some bands thick, some thin. In the north and central areas of California, zigzag lines, and all throughout California, horizontal and radiating lines around the mouth and cheeks, were prevalent.

Ceremonial marking of the flesh (tattooing) was done with available regional materials. Stones, such as obsidian, flint, and quartz were used throughout the North. The Pomo used a bone from the the foreleg of a squirrel. Porcupine quills were used by some Northeast groups, especially the Achomawi and Atsugewi. In the East-Central area, pine needles were used and in the arid regions cactus thorns were used. The Pomo used poison oak sap to increase the intensity of the welts. A mixture of coal and grease was used by Yokuts and red mineral pigment was used by the Pomo. Tattooing amongst the Indians marked adulthood and a measured "dentalia" (recorded wealth). It was used for medicine (tattooing over painful areas) and attaining supernatural powers for talismanic reasons.

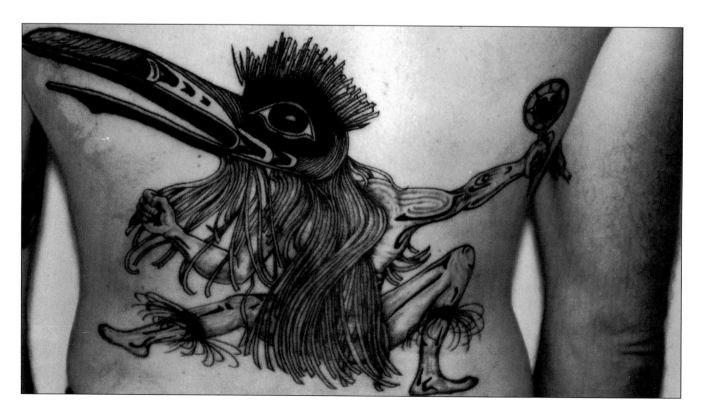

ODE TO THE BLACKFOOT TRIBE

"Tattooed on my arm is a picture of the Keepers of Nature. Deep in my veins these Indian men have hidden in my blood. I have given them life by choosing them as tattoo.

They must be free… to roam… to ride. With my forefathers on my arm, and the Blackfoot Mountains in the background. I can stand tall. As high as the sky. They give me Love. They give me pride."

—Ron Baker,
Blackfoot Indian

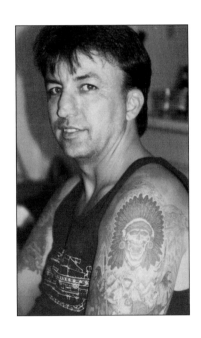

"I wanted to carry on the other side of my heart… The colors of my altar as they sit representing the directions, the buffalo sits in the center of the circle, the buffalo, the provider, the protector, the giver of all life."

— Wakian Luta
Bluza, Roger Broer, Lakota
Oglala Tribe, Artist

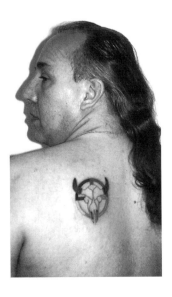

"I am an American Indian, and a physician on a reservation in Northern Idaho. Mad Dog is what I think Medical Doctor stands for. The dog depicts the typical reservation dog and the war bonnet represents my heritage.

BETTER RED THAN DEAD, is a satire on BETTER DEAD THAN RED & THE ONLY GOOD INDIAN IS A DEAD INDIAN. Red is for my race, not my politics.

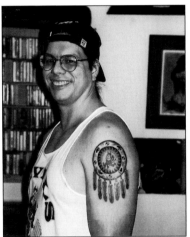

The war-shield protects the warrior as well as providing a way to express the symbolism that is important to that warrior. It is made of buffalo rawhide and willow and can repel arrows and bullets.

Red and black are my colors and they encircle the shield. The four colored circles represent the medicine wheels with the colors representing a color of a direction… east, west, etc.

The bear is a symbol of the power of healing and since I am a physician, the medicine wheels and bear prints are significant. The seven eagle feathers give power and represent the seven spiritual directions; creator, sky, father, earth mother and the four winds.

The devil has several meanings in Indian culture. There is no evil force or Satan figure, so the concept of the devil is not part of our culture. Personally for me it has meaning. This devil is from Arizona State University, where I went to college and launched my medical career. Also in the third grade I was the

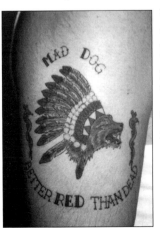

unanimous choice for a mischievous devil in a play — my public performing debut. He was as playful and mischievous as I am. The sun is for Sun Devil as well as an important part of Indian religion — Sun Dancing."

— Doctor David Baines
Tlingit/Tsiwpsian
Coeur D'Alene

MY TOTEMIC BACKPIECE

"I CHOSE AN AMERICAN INDIAN theme for my backpiece because it reminds me of a time when there were not so many differences in the world. The people and all living and non-living things were one. Their survival depended on it.

"These totems lend me the powers of my personal spirit guides and I wear them proudly. The word 'totem' is from the Chippewa language 'ototeman,' meaning 'his brother and sister,' or kin.

"By wearing an animal totem I can contact the very essence of all that is the spirit of that particular animal.

"The power of my totem animal can draw me into complete harmony with the strength of that particular animal. But this can only happen if I am willing to let it happen, and willing to learn the lessons of life that my spirit guides can teach me.

"Here is a look at the primary power of my totems:

1. **Deer:** speed, quick thinking, acute hearing with a gentleness of spirit that can heal all wounds. Lesson: *Don't push others hard, be accepting.*

2. **Hawk:** A hunter's totem; aggressive, observant. Lesson: *Be aware of signs in life, notice, receive, act if needed.*

3. **Cougar:** Another hunter's totem. Invulnerable, able to find lost things, power to heal, protective, leadership. Lesson: *Use power of leadership wisely, without insisting others follow. Roar with conviction, power and laughter.*

4. **Wolf:** Wolf is a teacher, gives and interprets. Lesson: *As long as you continue to learn, life goes on.*

"At the base of my back lies Grandmother Earth. She being the beginning of all life. She wears a symbolic red head wrap. Red is the color of the East, the beginning of life.

"To my right is 'Eagle Woman,' who brings the powers and talents of a medicine woman to my story. On my left side is a woman who has fallen asleep at her daily tasks, and rests her head on her basket. Perhaps she dreams of animal totems or maybe she seeks advice from spirits in her dream world. Remember, the American Indian's life was controlled by their dreams.

"Whenever decisions were to be made they consulted their dreams."

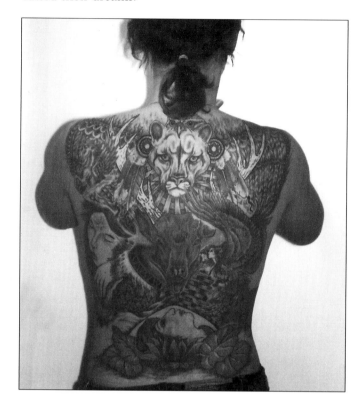

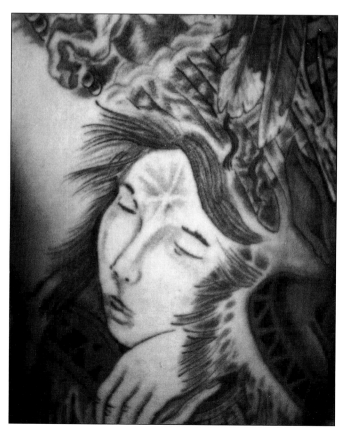

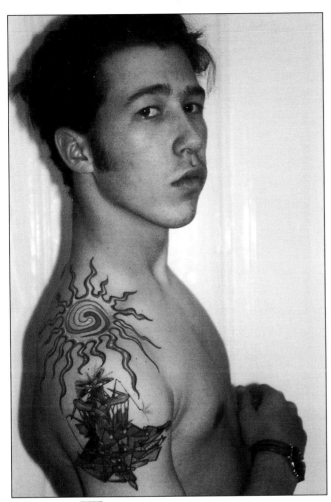

VOICE WITHIN

DAVID ARCHULETTA is a bright man in his twenties. He studies rhetoric at UC Berkeley, and is from Mendocino. He comes from a creative family; his mother, Susan Archuletta is a gifted musician. He and his brothers and sister come from a long line of artists and musicians.

David was raised in a Sufi Community in the 70's, living in Morocco, Pakistan and in Europe. Being of Mescalito-Apache heritage as well as Eastern European Transylvanian and Basque gypsy... out of his unconscious rose these images that he chose as tattoos in honor of his heritage.

Tattoo images are a dynamic force in relationship to the wearer and the world. They are honed in a subrosian manner, rising out of the unconscious like a sprouting seed from fertile ground. They are expressive of that very moment extracted from a lifetime, and lasting for the duration, capsulized in time and imprinted with ink permanently onto the wearer's skin. Here are reflections from David Archuletta's "Voice Inside."

"We are finally beginning to find our lost spirits, our forgotten tribal families. I am part Mescalito-Apache Indian. This heritage is an integral part of my being. Though the culture of that people is physically extinct, I still feel the spirit of it inside me wherever I go, whatever I do."

"When I finally saw the image that I wanted as a tattoo, it was like an open circle had been closed. The image in my mind fit the image before me like two halves of a whole; it was a key going into a door, food filling my stomach, air filling my lungs. Staring at the image was like staring at a reflection of myself. It reflected what no mirror could reflect; my soul."

"My tattoo speaks to me. It is a strong voice sent out from the depths of my inner-self. The voice is powerful and is in a language that no tongue can speak. It is the language of the Image. My tattoo says what I cannot put into words. It presents a part of me to the world that cannot be described in any other way but ritual and image. When I show people my tattoo, I see pure fascination in their eyes. I see that they, too, have something inside of them that calls for 'release and recognition.'

"When I had my image permanently tattooed on my body, I recognized something that has been for a long time internal. When the internal image reached the outside body, a permanent channel was established between my conscious and subconscious; mind and body; world and self. Being tattooed is taking a special place inside your heart and recognizing it to yourself and the world. It is like speaking what is in your soul."

When we ink our skins with totems of our choosing, we connect ourselves to the ancient world with these images breathing within us. It is through our flesh that we can express this cross-cultural art vision as a statement without a political power play. Along with this committed expression is a link of the mind to the body. As in the case of David Archuletta, it can be a spiritually enriching experience. This ink, under the third layer of our skin, clearly states that the wearer has undergone an act of communion.

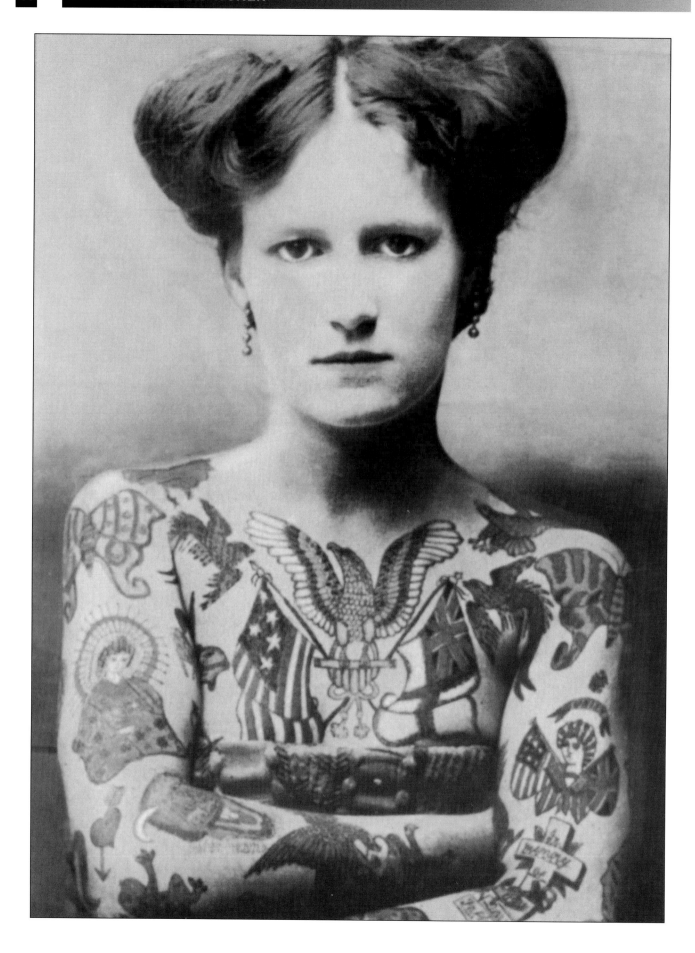

TATTOOED WOMEN IN CIRCUS SIDESHOWS

THE TATTOOED LADIES in traveling circuses, sideshows and carnivals were part of an alien subculture called Freaks. The "performers" developed the closeness of a family; bred of long hours, constant traveling and the struggle to survive. The tattooed lady existed on the border of public and private, aberrant and acceptable, conspicuous and discreet. She made herself accessible to the curious crowds who paid their fare to see her as a sideshow spectacle. She has profited financially and historically in the tattoo world.

Throughout our lives we are inspired by images, acts, public figures and philosophies. I was inspired by these tattooed women who are individual traveling art galleries. They have inspired me to realize my freedom to express my individuality, and to live proudly with my tattooed skin. A few exotic names: Astoria, Princess Cristina, Miss Gypsy Castella, Saharet, Queenie Morris from Ireland, Alexia from Australia, Ethella, Lyda Akado from Germany, Angora, Astra and La Belle Irene from France are just a few of many whose colorful lives have inspired me and many others.

I am forty-six years of age. My grandmother is ninety-one. We talk often on the phone. During one conversation she asked me if I was "preparing for my future." I told her that I live so much in the present, and that I wasn't.

At the time, I was researching material for our Tattoo Museum which features tattooed people from circus sideshows. That evening, as I was getting ready for bed, I happened to look at my reflection in the full length mirror with another set of eyes. I realized then that, unconsciously, I was indeed preparing myself for the future by tattooing my body. And just perhaps, when I am old and white-haired, wearing coke-bottle glasses, I will be seen dancing through the shopping malls in a tutu, singing a little song, showing off my tattoos, and then passing around my leopard skin pillbox hat! Who knows what the future will hold?

History holds a wealth of information for us to draw upon and share with each other. Here are a few stories of women in circus sideshows.

At the impressionable age of fourteen, Artoria Gibbons, a Wisconsin farm girl, ran away from home into the arms of Charles "Red" Gibbons.

Red was a tattooist in the circus, and he tattooed an angel on Artoria's wrist, which was the beginning of her career as a circus sideshow attraction under the name Artoria. She was a staunch Baptist who looked like a school marm. She and Red married and traveled with Ringling Brothers. Her tattoos were religiously inspired, and she felt through her tattoos she was preparing herself for the "Heavenly Kingdom." She chose "respectable" designs for her tapestry, such as a portrait of Baby Jesus on her left thigh and the Madonna on her right. She had Botticelli's Annunciation on her left arm and Raphael's Angels on her shoulder. Michelangelo's Holy Family was tattooed on her biceps and a portrait of George Washington was proudly displayed between her breasts. Red tattooed his own portrait on her as a statement of ownership and advertisement of his tattooing skills.

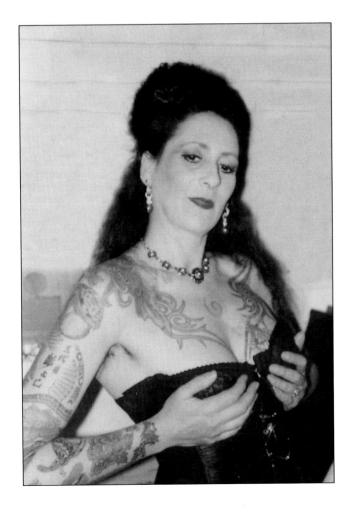

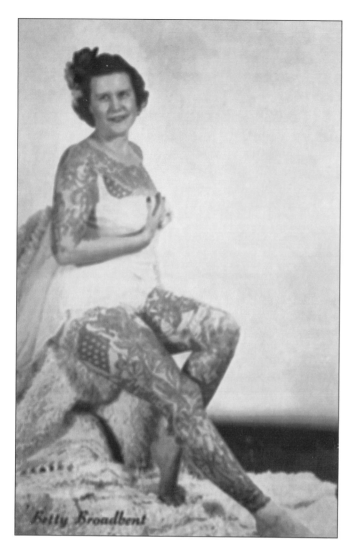

Betty Broadbent

many circus performers. It was in 1927 that Betty was offered a contract to be the youngest tattooed woman in the world for Ringling Brothers. She also rode jump horses and bucking mules. She became a tattoo artist in New York and Montreal for a time during the 1930s. She also worked independently in shows in Australia and New Zealand from 1937 to 1939. Her last circus performance was in 1967 with Clyde Beatty. In August, 1981, she became the first member of San Francisco Tattoo Art Museum's Hall of Fame at Lyle Tuttle's. She later moved to Florida and raised small show animals, rare species of chickens, dogs and rabbits.

Annetta Nerona, was a German sideshow performer. She wore tattoos of portraits of Goethe, Schiller, Emperor Wilhelm II and Richard Wagner. Lady Viola was another who had tattoos of six U.S. presidents, Babe Ruth and Charlie Chaplin.

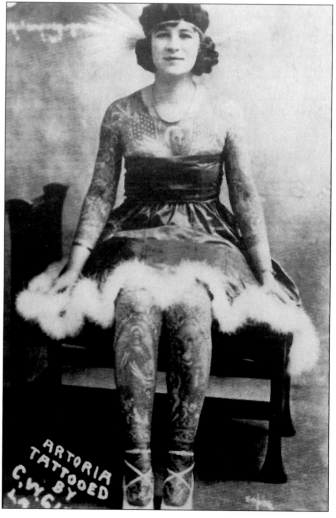

ARTORIA TATTOOED BY C.W.G.

There were several tattooed women running the circuits of carnivals and circuses at the turn of the century. La Belle Irene was adorned with tattoos of angels, butterflies, flowers and inscriptions such as "Nothing without Labor," and "Never Despair." It was with and through her that draping scrolls came to be popular in American tattooing. She fabricated mysterious tales about her tattoos, such as being abducted by savages. These tales were part of her show, which added intrigue.

Betty Broadbent was another well known tattooed sideshow attraction during the late 1920s. It all started for her when she was baby-sitting a neighbor's child and wandered down the boardwalk. She was so impressed and intrigued that a couple of years later she took her savings to New York where most of her 364 tattoos were done by famed artist Charlie Wagner, who tattooed

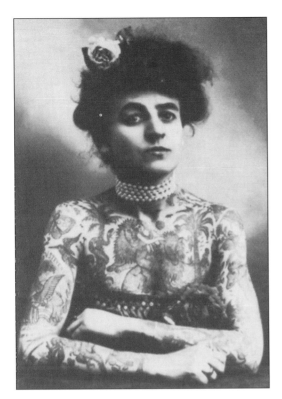

The tattooed women in circus sideshows during the late 1940s to 1950s were "Performance Artists," as well as living canvases of art. These women were instrumental in the historical moment when art was liberated from the art galleries, studios and museums, and put on public exhibit in the traveling sideshows.

History repeats itself in mysterious ways. Plan for your future. Get heavily tattooed.

Be Art with a Pulse, dancing in the shopping malls.

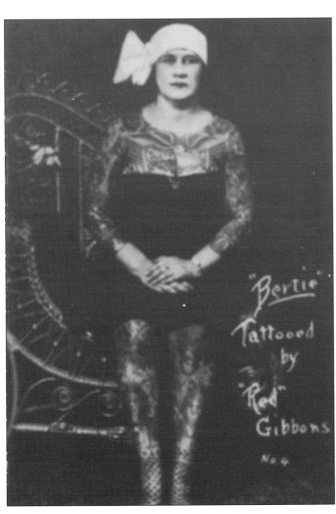

"Bertie"
Tattooed
by
"Red"
Gibbons
No. 4

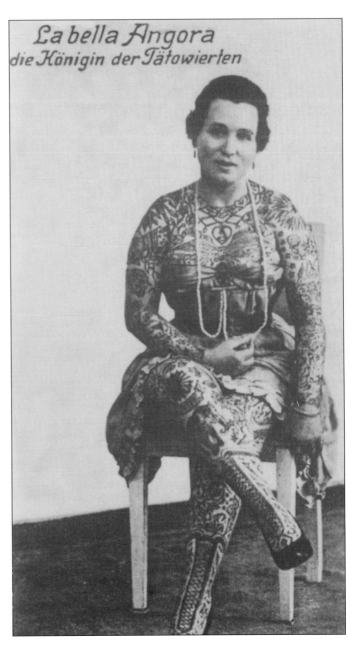

La bella Angora
die Königin der Tätowierten

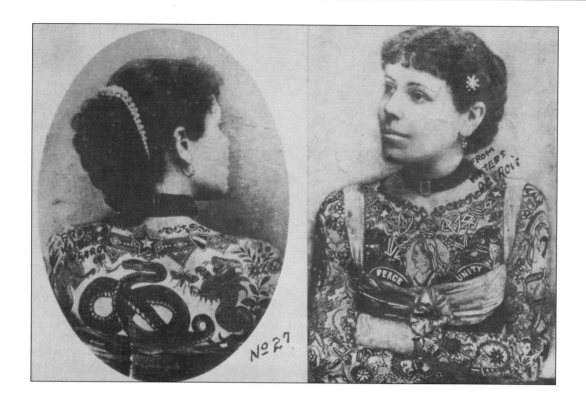

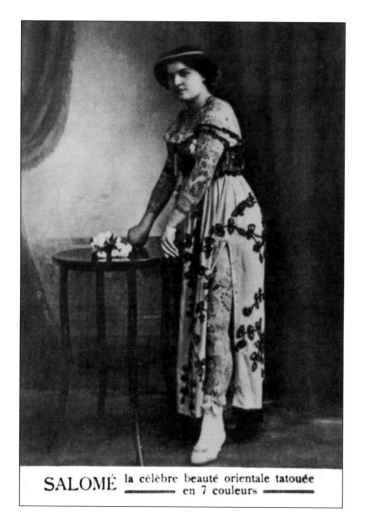

SALOMÉ la célèbre beauté orientale tatouée
en 7 couleurs

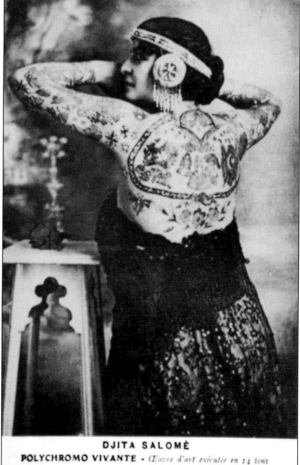

DJITA SALOMÉ
POLYCHROMO VIVANTE - Œuvre d'art exécutée en 14 tons
Par les Peaux Rouges de DAKOTA (U. S.)

CAPTAIN DON LESLIE
"MR. SIDESHOW"

For ten years people have been coming into our Main Street Tattoo Studio, and their first question has always been, "Does it hurt?" But now it is, "Who is Captain Don?" This question is asked in reference to the festive circus sideshow atmosphere they see: the colorful billboards with fire-eaters, sword swallowers and elephants, extravagant sequined costumes, sensational photographs and historical folk art that decorate the walls.

Captain Don Leslie, known as Mr. Sideshow, is a sword swallower, fire-eater, human blockhead, musician and tattooed circus man. He is also our mentor in addition to being a generous contributor to Triangle Tattoo History Museum. His display gives us valuable insight into the history of the circus sideshow and tattooing. His portrait in full regalia is shown here. One wing of the museum features his background; memorabilia from forty-two years of his circus life cover the walls, ceiling to floor. His display is surrounded by photographs of his predecessors, the Tattooed People of the Circus Sideshow.

Last week Captain Don phoned us to report his recent performance in Chico. I asked him how it went. "Well, Chinchilla, it was OK. Only one person went down when I did my human blockhead act." (Meaning, when he hammered a spike into his nose, only one person passed out.) "Does that happen often?" I asked. "Yes," he said, "At the circus people come to stuff themselves with popcorn, cotton candy and corn dogs. Then they ride the roller coaster, and when that's over, they wander into the sideshow tent where I swallow my swords and eat fire or do my blockhead act, and four to ten people go down during the performance. It's very hot in the big tops."

Recently Captain Don was in our living room. He was here to continue the video interview of him for his biography, *He Who Lives By The Sword Is Always Broke*. Being anything but ordinary, his life story is fascinating, raw and glorious.

The unspoken motto by which the circus folk live is, FIRST THE CIRCUS, THEN GOD, THE FLAG & THE COUNTRY. Just as the cowboy waters his horse before himself, or the soldier puts his country before his own life, the circus folks put the circus before anything else. This proved true when, in a 1989 Seattle performance, Captain Don told us, "The circus always came first, even when my sword slipped

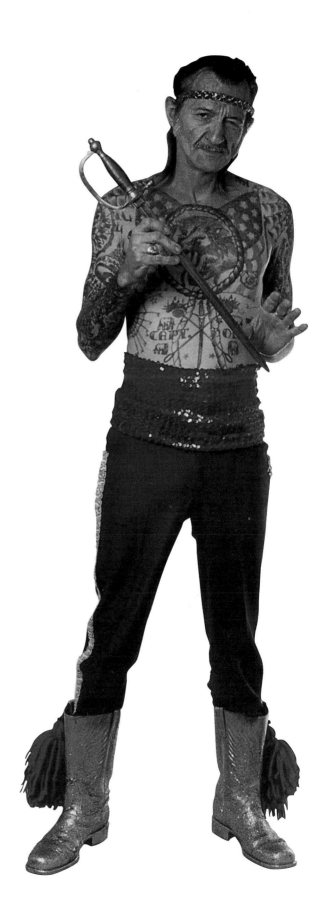

and cut my esophagus and I was hemorrhaging. I still finished my performance."

He is a quiet man. When he stays with us, we hardly know he is here. He sets up studio on our divan, surrounded by his books, paints, brushes, and the crumbs from the cheddar cheese crackers he loves to nibble. When he is not on the divan, we find him with his nose in the file cabinets in which his past is being preserved. He is also a fisherman. He doesn't care if he catches fish. He just enjoys the meditation of the beautiful outdoors.

An avid reader, Captain Don can converse on almost any subject. He can recite famous quotations for hours. He knows the lyrics to so many songs that he is also referred to as

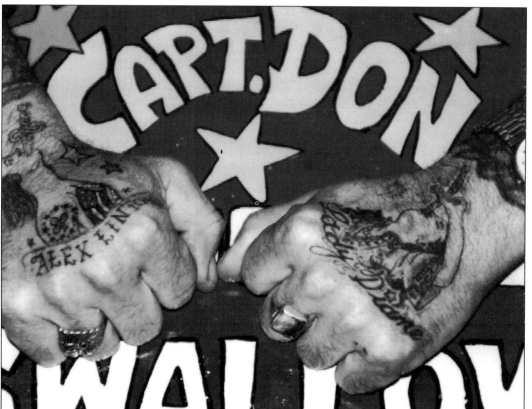

glowing through his chest!). In his street performance days in San Francisco, Boston and New Orleans, he sometimes swallowed a bayonet ten times an hour, five hours a day — which is fifty times a day for six days in a row. . . count that during a forty-two year period of time!

Mr. G. and I were honored when Captain Don asked us to tattoo the backs of his hands. I tattooed Alex Linton (his mentor) on his right hand. Mr. G. tattooed Lady Diane (his protégé) on the other. A postcard of his hands was produced and is available from the Tattoo Archives in Berkeley, California.

A portrait of Captain Don as The Seven of Swords is on a tarot deck from the 80s. He is swallowing five swords and holding two, one in each hand. Other noted people are also depicted in this deck. The designer's name was Maud and she was from Berkeley. We are looking for the deck, so if anyone out there in reading land knows of this deck of tarot cards, please contact us.

In April, Captain Don was contacted by the Discovery Channel and flown First Class to L.A. for an in-depth interview for a documentary film on the history of American circus sideshows. They had a list of 290 names of perform-

Captain Don, Man of 5000 Songs. When he sings to an audience, he will yell out to them, "Call out a song I don't know and get a drink on the house." He has written twenty-five songs and has put out a record album as well.

In his lifetime, he has swallowed a staggering number of swords. In the circus sideshow, he would do 18-22 performances a day. During each performance, he would swallow fifteen times: either a bayonet, knife, sword, a saber, oil dipstick, a screwdriver, or a lit florescent tube (which one could see

ers, freaks, owners and operators of the sideshows during the last century, but only twenty-four people were contacted for interviews.

Captain Don Leslie is still performing. Due to the extinction of the sideshow, he performs in nightclubs and halls. Come up to our Museum and view his life and history.

He is available for performances
and can be reached through the Triangle Tattoo Museum.

MODERN DAY TRIBAL RITUALS

NEW TRIBALISM IS an emerging art form. It is directly influenced by the Dyak, Iban, Samoan and Maori people of the South Sea Islands. These designs, bold, black, sculptural adapt well to the natural curves of the human body and are used as tattoo designs. They are impressive on fabric and pottery as well.

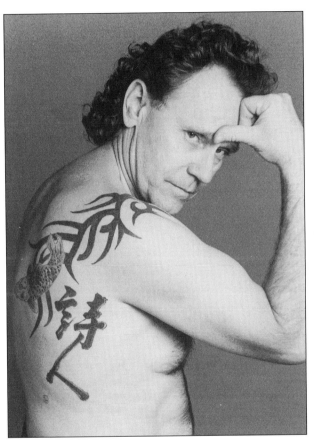

I was introduced to tribal tattoos 17 years ago in American Samoa. The occasion was the opening of the first American Samoan Bank. I was on a South Sea tour with my mother. There was a festive ceremony in the square adjoining the mahogany dock. An American ship brought in one million dollars for the opening. We watched the tribal chiefs, stately and corpulent, walk to their appointed seats under the shade of a banyan tree. I got my first fascinating glimpse of tribal tattoos. Jet black linear designs were visible from mid-waist to knee. These tattoos mark their ancestry and are a ritualistic part of their culture.

There is a significant re-emergence of what is called the "Modern Primitive." This is seen in art, culture and tattoos. I am one of the many Modern Primitives. Just the other morning, after my shower, I caught a glimpse of my tribal tattooed bodice in the foggy morning mirror. This vision shifted me back in time to the memory of my introduction to tribal tattoos. I am wearing designs influenced by the Samoan chiefs. At that time, when I first saw them I never would have imagined that I would now be studying the symmetry of my own tribal tattoos, or be a tattoo artist, tattooing those very designs under the third layer of people's skin.

Ron Salisbury (pictured) is another Modern Primitive. He describes himself as a "male, WASP, middle class, bourgeois banker." This is his statement:

"The long two and a half hour ride home was something magical. First, the winding road through the dark redwoods into the inland valley, my right shoulder stiff and burning, something pushing out like a benevolent alien grabbing its first few breaths. I felt special, unique. This feeling was something that had been missing. It had to do with the feeling that if there had been no pain, then the tattoo on my shoulder might as well have been house paint. I passed through the millennial pain of ritual. And this tied me to some Sioux or Mandan hanging from tethers; some Micronesian stretched on a mat in the shade, gritting his teeth, maybe whimpering as his spirit was pricked into his legs for hours. Pain and history seem tied together. I feel what one does is ritualistically abrade the skin over the spot where a mark already existed. This which rose through my muscle and psyche, had always been there, and you, Chinchilla, served as the Shaman waving your wand or medicine pouch. A guide like Castaneda's Don Juan. And I did the rest."

And so this is a modern day ritual of a primitive act. A necessary primitive act. Sacrosanct and profound. Enduring. Self satisfying.

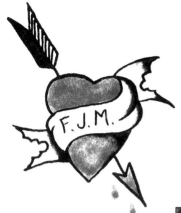

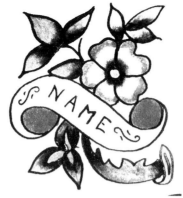

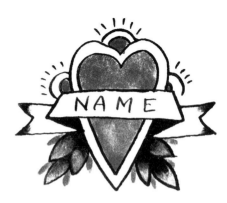

EVERY X-MAS,
OUR STUDIO OFFERS
A 15% DISCOUNT
FOR TAKING THE
EX OUTTA X-MAS.

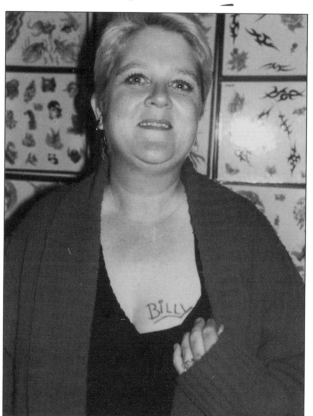

THINK
BEFORE
YOU INK

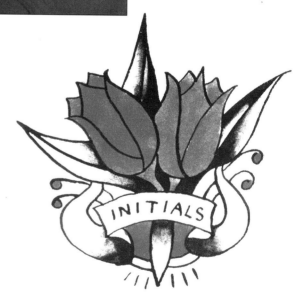

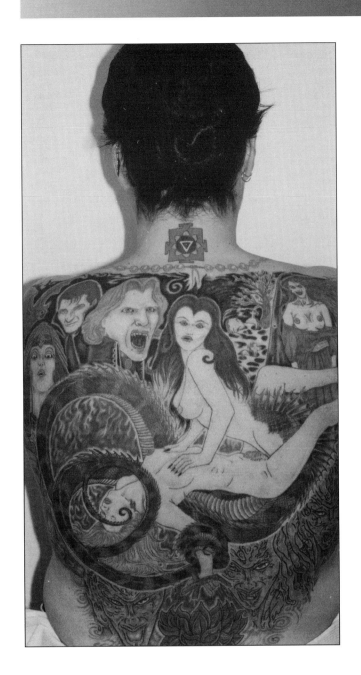

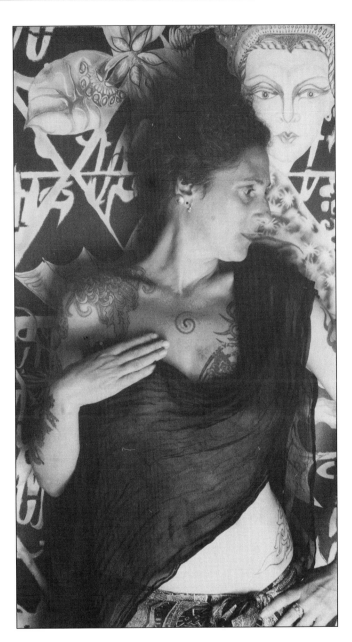

"The tattoo artist initiates the ceremonial process with the person wanting the tattoo. Even though there are no drums beating or chanting this is perhaps the oldest ritual on earth."

— Mr. G.

TATTOOS: DO THEY HURT?

IN RESPONSE TO THIS QUESTION, I was asked to tattoo HELL YES on the inside of a tattoo artist's lower lip. This was the strangest request I've ever had, and I complied, because no one else within a 150-mile radius knew how to do it. This is the most unusual tattoo I have ever done, and have been kissing that very lip for eight years. It belongs to the love of my life.

There is a T-shirt that has HELL YES! IT HURTS

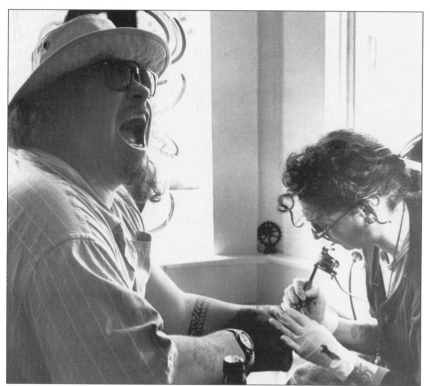

in bold letters on the front. But tattooing as it is done nowadays is not as primitive as in the past, when blunt needles and thick pigments were pushed under the flesh in a brutal manner, and a heavy scab with pain was an integral part of the process.

With any new experience, such as a new job, losing your virginity, your first driving test, date, etc., the apprehension is more traumatic than the actual event.

Does it hurt? Well, it is a bit shocking at first, as it is electric, hot and stinging, but is not down-right painful unless it is on a bone such as the elbow, knee or spine. Different parts of the body have varying sensitivi-

ty. Tattooing is a rite of passage, but not as radical as circumcision, childbirth, scarification or the piercing of the tongue. Some people describe it as irritating, or like a cat scratch, but mostly it is a hot sensation with a slight bite to it. Tattoos are minor abrasions, less than skinning your knee, and instead of getting a scar, you get a colorful and meaningful design of your choice.

Our bodies are miraculous organisms, installed with automatic responses. One of these is the releasing of endorphines. As a person receives a tattoo, their body releases endorphines and floods them with a feeling of euphoria, similar to a runner's high. This may be one of the many factors that make tattoos so appealing. Tattoos are like potato chips, kisses, chocolates, small victories: We want to repeat the experience again and again. Just look at us and our customers. Most people who get one tattoo come back for more. Tattoos are an expression of our freedom, our indelible commitment to the moment and our future. We wear our dreams, aspirations, beliefs proudly, like a medal or a fine piece of jewelry. Our bodies are the ultimate canvas for art.

Here are a few other things to keep in mind when you go for your tattoo:

Look for a clean environment. Ask around and get references before getting a tattoo. Check on the shop's reputation. Look at some of their healed tattoos. Ask if their needles are new. Ask to look at a portfolio of their tattoos. Consider the presentation. If you feel good about everything after the initial look around…go for it!

There are many things to consider when getting a tattoo, especially for women. Think about social situations you might be in where your tattoo would show, like at a cocktail party, or the country club, or another country where there might be prejudice about tattooing. Do you want to have the option of being able to hide it? Because, remember, wherever you go, your tattoo goes with you!

Be Art With A Pulse! It's O.K.

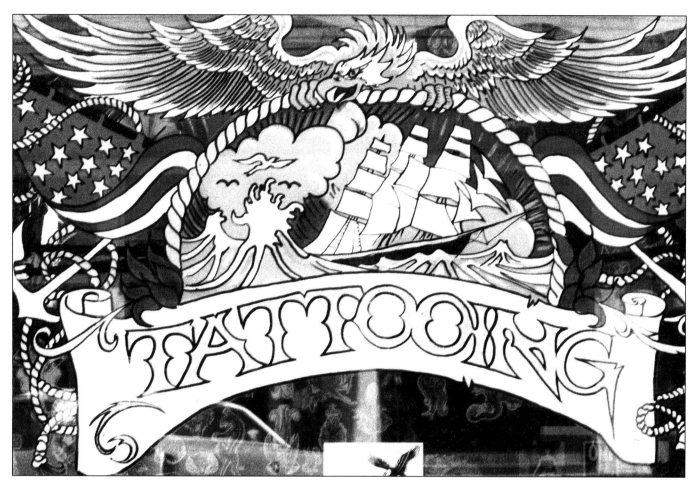

BART BIRD

IT WAS ONE OF THOSE cold windy nights on Laurel Street in downtown Fort Bragg. Our sign was blowing at a right angle which meant the gusts were at 30mph. The shop sounded like a beehive, with three tattoo machines buzzing away at 100 mph, pushing dreams and ink under the flesh and into the psyche of three people. It was warm and cozy inside, filled to the max with customers and their support groups. The smell of green soap and pizza were in the air.

I was finishing up a winged dragon on a man's biceps, highlighting its eyes and claws… when a cocky, slightly sauced young man walked in, bringing with him a refreshing gust of cold sea air. I looked up from my dragon, the color purple dripping off the point of my needles and asked if I could help him with anything. "Yes," he said, "I want a tattoo of Bart Simpson on a skateboard with red shoes giving the bird. " "What kind

of bird?" I asked. "You know, The Bird, the Bird! The Middle Finger."

He was growing impatient with me and I was enjoying it. It is fun to be a woman dealing with a young man's tattoo request. I told him that he was a nice looking young man and I couldn't possibly put Bart Simpson giving The Bird on him, that he was not a bathroom wall and I would feel like I would be defacing him. I ended our conversation by telling him that I was old enough to be his mother and I wouldn't even put The Bird on my own son, but I would ask one of the other artists if they would. So I turned around and asked "Hey, Steven, do you want to tattoo The Bird on Bart Simpson?" "Hell, yes!" he replied.

So I tattooed all but The Bird on Bart, and Steven tattooed The Bird. The young man looked at his finished tattoo and looked at me, smiled and said, "That's Bad!"I looked at him and said "Bad?" He said in an exasperated voice, "Look Chinchilla, Bad is good and Good is bad, get it?"

MY MOM IS GOING TO KILL ME WHEN SHE SEES THIS TATTOO

THIS IS A COMMON PHRASE uttered while under the buzz of the tattoo needles for the first time. We usually respond with, "Don't tell her who did this to you!" The Mom's-gonna-kill-me statement is so commonly heard in different languages and tattoo studios worldwide that a tattoo t-shirt is on the market that reads: *My Mom Is Going To Kill Me When She Sees This Tattoo.*

But this phrase was not uttered with the Machado family from Ceres, California. They are now a tattooed family of six. This includes mom, dad, and their four kids. The daughter asks, "Mom, look at the beautiful color for my orchid, what do you think, should it be lighter?" Mom responds, "It's perfect for you, your colors, go for it." The Machado family is one of many who come to Fort Bragg for their "tattoo vacations." This is their sixth visit this year. On their daughter's 18th birthday, mother and daughter got matching roses. On their next visit they got butterflies. Dad got a big tiger on his back, another on his arm and yet another on his thigh. This colorful family are part of the New Age Tattoo Renaissance.

Usually when an offspring begins his or her journey to adulthood, it is to separate from the parents. It is arduous, rebellious, and curiously liberating. Most often parents are not supportive and accepting. But nowadays, more and more families are sharing this journey together, creating this avenue for expressing their individuality with pleasure and acceptance. This is happening via the ancient art of tattooing.

We humans need rituals to connect us to one another, and to our culture in celebration of life's passages. Birth, circumcision, baptism, graduation, birthdays, marriages

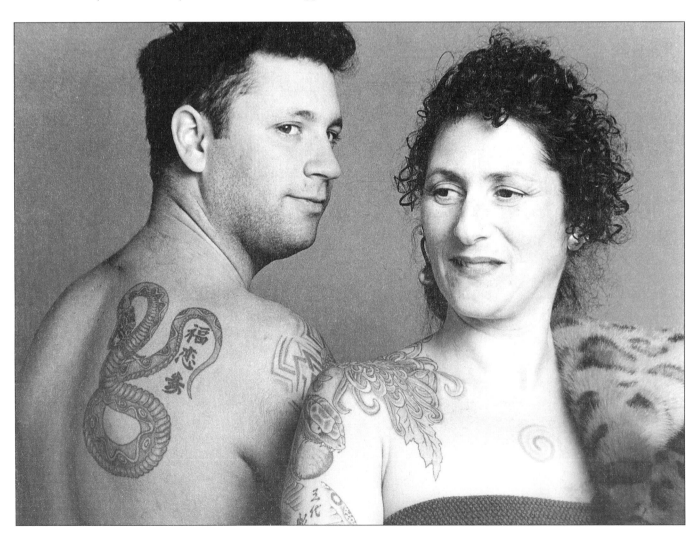

and funerals are a few of them. These rituals did not include marking one's self with symbols like tribal cultures did for centuries... until recently. My son, Mr. G. and I each have matching Horiyoshi snakes on our bodies. A man walked into Triangle Tattoo, looked around and asked, "Why do you people get these tattoos?" Mr. G. looked up at him from the tiger he was tattooing and said, "Because we are a Lost Culture searching for symbols."

All cultures express themselves with symbols. We create them, borrow them from other cultures, weave them, eat, paint and draw them, chant and write them, and also wear them as tattooed images under the third layer of our skins. Our choices are reflections of who we are and how we relate to the world. We compose ourselves with and from these symbols like an eclectic tapestry. Being a pleasure oriented society includes the appreciation and need of self adornment and feeling of bonding with one another and the world. Here are some stories of these bondings within the family structure.

A father and daughter who reunited after 32 years came in to celebrate their reunion with a tattoo. She got a red heart with Dad tattooed on her right arm and he got her name, Truth, tattooed on his right arm in Japanese calligraphy.

One couple wrote a letter to us expressing their feelings about their new tattoos: "This might sound corny, but our tattoo experience brought us closer to one another."
Sonya & Andrew

A woman told us that her mother said to her, "Nothing can ever rob you of your joy." So in a stressful time of her life, she came in for the tattoo of a hummingbird that she had painted, which symbolizes joy for her. She left feeling joyous, saying "This hummingbird on my shoulder is a symbol I will always have with me, reminding me of my mother's words, and I feel stronger now."

A jolly woman dressed in her nurse's uniform, red-eyed from working the graveyard shift at the hospital walked in with her three sons. They came for their Christmas tattoos. They got matching calligraphy which symbolized their last name. Their father was lost in the war, and this was a bonding ceremony for them as a family.

The mother of two daughters walked in with them, one crying because she was too young to get a tattoo, and the other excited to get her tattoo of an anklet, a gold chain with a charm of her astral sign for her 18th birthday. The mother already had several tattoos and while waiting for her daughter, discussed the design of her next one. We had to console the younger daughter, suggesting she get some good removable tattoos and put them in different places on her body, so that in four years she will know exactly what she wants and where she wants it. We told her we'd be happy to tattoo her when she was of age. She wondered if her tattoo would show up with all of her freckles. She said her mother told her that she was kissed by the fairies. We told her that her freckles were her natural tattoos.

A local family of eight have all been here for tattoos. The parents who are in their seventies came in first, then their children and eventually, when of age, their grandchildren. They all support each other's individuality with their tattoos.

"I want to incorporate the names of my children and grandchildren into the beautiful image that I will carry with me throughout this life. My daughter Christina and I are going to get our tattoos at the same time to deepen and strengthen the meaning." These are the sentiments of June, an artist in our community.

Gloria, a local artist-weaver, and her sons Sean and Joshua, both poets, have designed and received several tattoos. Here is a poem Gloria wrote:

Family Tattooed

Inward character placed on outer layer...
for permanent viewing
We choose symbols of who we are and what we see...
Inside ourselves, Spirit revealed.
Like coming out of hiding. Each one of us different,
unique and bold enough to say... See...
this is who I am. We stand united in our
individuality... tattooed-marked
Smiling... Close to each other. Family.

TATTOOED STATEMENTS:
VISUAL AND LITERAL

IN THIS CENTURY, UNLIKE any other, many profound statements will be seen tattooed on people's bodies, i.e.: FREEDOM TO BREED WILL BRING RUIN TO ALL… (This was the request of a 19 year old girl, and is now tattooed in turquoise blue letters around a pure white lily on her slender ankle.)

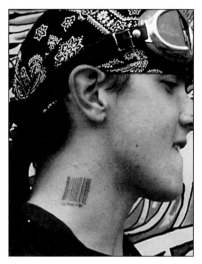

The words NO CODE BLUE will be found tattooed on the chest, over the heart of people who may end up in a trauma unit. This means "Leave me alone. Do not interfere. Let me die!" We have tattooed this mostly on trauma care workers.

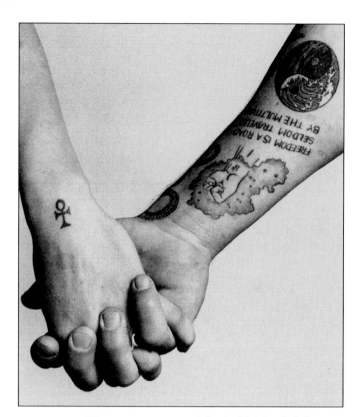

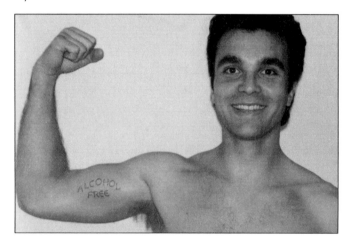

FREEDOM IS A ROAD SELDOM TRAVELED BY THE MULTITUDES, WHAT DOES NOT KILL ME MAKES ME STRONGER, BORN TO BE FREE, BAD TO THE BONE, are commonly tattooed statements. The words YOUTH GONE WILD next to a pair of flaming purple tennis shoes adorn a young woman's arm.

The statements DRUG FREE and STRAIGHT EDGE will be found tattooed across the broad shoulders of young men. They are in two-inch high Old English letters, celebrating their sobriety . Many AA'ers and NAer's celebrate their sobriety with the adornment of tattoos. One woman wears a series of colorful roses like a fabulous bouquet winding up her arm.

A Danish bicyclist rode in to have the words NO JUSTICE NO PEACE inscribed on his tanned shoulders. The words LOVE & HATE are found tattooed on the hands of young hoodlums.

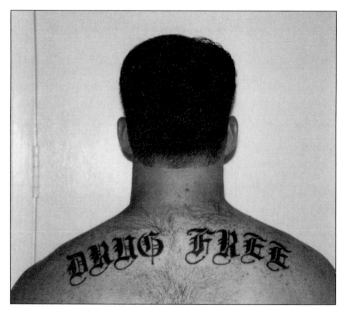

One very interesting man has the words HELL YES tattooed on the inside of his lower lip, so when he is old and in a retirement home and the the nurse asks him if he would like his medication, all he has to do is roll his lip down and she'll know that he wants it! Soon the tattoo HELL NO will be tattooed on the inside of his upper lip, so when the nurse asks him if he wants his enema now, he can just roll that lip up and she will get the the message!

One day a young man came to us and I asked, "May I help you?" He replied, "Yes, I would like YOUR NAME on my butt." Shocked but trying to remain cool, I replied, "But you don't even know me. Why would you want my name on your butt?" He said, "Because that is what I want." At that point I thought he was very strange, excused myself for a moment and went to get Mr. G., told him what was happening. He rolled up his sleeves and

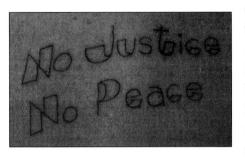

went out to ask this man what he wanted and got the same reply. After a few moments, we realized he wanted exactly what he asked for the words YOUR NAME on his butt. Well, he got it and paid for it in ten minutes by making bets at the closest bar by saying to someone, "I bet you $5 that I have YOUR NAME tattooed on my butt!"

Another man got the words, "Girls, Girls, Girls"

and others have the words YOU ALWAYS WIN WHEN YOU RIDE A HARLEY DAVIDSON TWIN, MAMA TRIED, TO THINE OWNSELF BE TRUE. The letters ALF meaning Animal Liberation Front are on a young man's forearm.

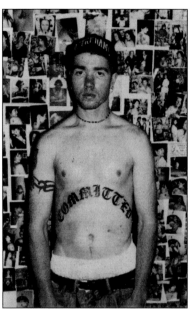

Along with the feeling of personal freedom, an explicit feeling of triumph is felt after receiving a tattoo. It is very powerful and fulfilling, as one realizes that through being tattooed, we connect ourselves to a wondrous and ancient world of tattoo.

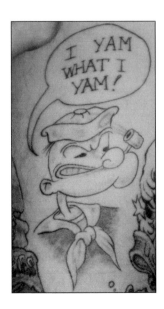

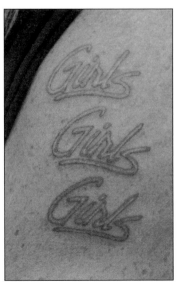

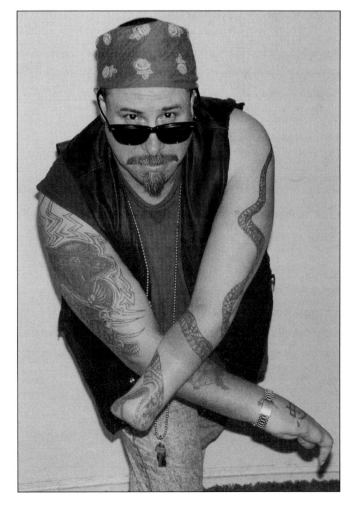

NEW AGE ICEMAN

TATTOOS ARE SOMETHING we can take with us everywhere we go. They will crawl into bed with us at night, accompany us in our dreams and wake up in the morning with us, staring out from our skins in the fogged morning mirror. They will follow us into our graves; perhaps later to be discovered, and provide a clue of our heritage.

Imagine 5,000 years from now. . . being exhumed from a vapor-lock in time and space, and on our mummified skins will be tattooed inscriptions of butterflies, dragons, skulls, castles, etc. What an exciting thought... to be associated to a tribe by our 20th century markings. Archeologists will discover the Dragon Tribe, The Tribe of Roses, Tribe of Skulls, and more. What an enigma we will be with the tattoos we carry with us from this century!

Many of us will be wearing tattoos of words and names: SAN FRANCISCO, FOREVER IN MY HEART SALLY, FUCK YOU, MAMA TRIED, MOM, DAD, BILLY, or MI LOCO VIDA (my crazy life), RIDE TO LIVE AND LIVE TO RIDE.

The recent discovery of The Iceman, a mummified Bronze-Age man in his 20's to 40's proved to history that tattooing has existed for more than 5,000 years, rather than the 2,500 years previously believed.

This 5,300-year-old Stone Age Wanderer was found lying intact, boots and all, preserved in a Similaun glacier high in the Alps near the border of Italy and Switzerland. He wore blue tattoos in the form of crosses and lines on his lower back, knees and ankle. The significance of his tattoos are still unknown, but they are a clue to the ancient civilization to which he belonged. There is speculation that perhaps he was a shaman.

Soon after the discovery of The Iceman, Robert D. Vinson came into Triangle Tattoo and Museum requesting the same markings as The Iceman. We did not have close-up illustrations but with the cooperation of National Geographic Magazine, Professor Dr. Konrad Spindler and Dr. Hans Moser of the Research Institute at the Leopold-Franzens Universitat of Innsbruck, I tattooed Mr. Vinson in December of 1993.

New discoveries such as these are evidence that tattooing is an integral element in most cultures of the world. Until recently, tattooing was rarely mentioned in university class rooms. To unveil this subject, one must dig deeply into hidden texts and studies, which have been eliminated from the general public's knowledge by fear and distaste.

Lost in the vaults of institutes and museums are yet more discoveries concerning ancient civilizations and their tattooed markings. Waiting silently for centuries in glaciers, enshrouded in tombs, buried in cities and caves are more glimpses of tattooed civilizations. When we are exhumed, what a diversified and puzzling dilemma we will present to historians and archeologists.

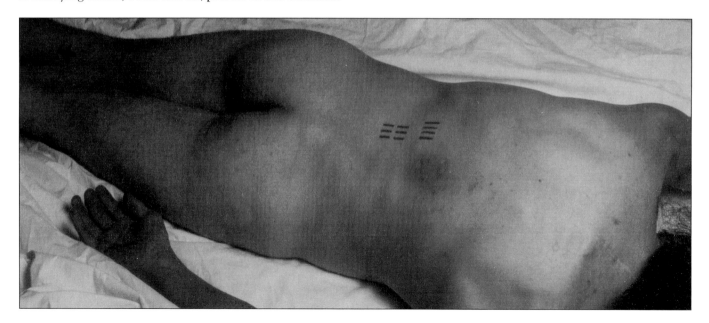

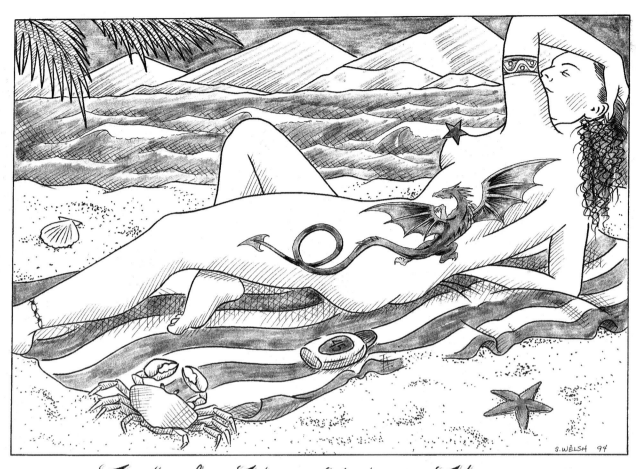

Wish You Were Here

EVEN TATTOOED PEOPLE GO ON VACATION

EVERYWHERE WE GO, there we are with our tattoos. Yes, even tattooed people go on vacations, sit on hot white sandy beaches, sip limone conagua purificado and margaritas, and eat greasy papas fritas, roasted camerones and fresh limey cerviche.

We went to Playa De Carmen on the Caribbean in Mexico. Bikini clad, we walked along the white sand into the turquoise blue water. All eyes shifted under reflector sunglasses. Whispers of, "Look at them" drifted our way in the tropical sea breeze. We were indeed curiosities. Like sideshow spectacles, yet no money was thrown our way.

There were three of us each immensely colorful with our many tattoos. What a collage we were against the white sand, the blue water. It was interesting and unnerving to be so exposed in a public place.

Under searing hot blue skies, we walked from our friends' casa in a coma-like trance down a white dirt road to the village square. Sweat poured from our bodies like long distance runners. I was afraid our tattoos would drip right off of us, like a watercolor painting in the rain. But instead, our tattoos begin their metamorphosis, started coming to life. The flowers on my arm and shoulder exuded a delicious scent and their petals threatened to fly off with the gentle breeze. There was an alchemic quality in the jungle… the mixture of greenery, humidity and the exotic song of the bird that made the tiger on

Mr. G.'s chest come to life and roar, stalking his prey. It seemed to want to spring from his chest and return to its home, the jungle. I had to hold him back.

The effect of the elements on our tattoos was significant. The tattooed prayers above our hearts seemed to rise from our skins, and became a chant to the approaching morning. The word MAGIC tattooed on my arm created the ambiance for all of this to happen. The Japanese Elvis on Mr. G.'s stomach took a refreshing dip in the sea. The flying corncob tattoo on his leg was roasted and ready to eat. His lucky lady, once lily white, was now golden brown. The pollywog tail swayed to and fro on his colorful arm as we swam in the ceynote, a sacred pool where virgins were once sacrificed. My water lily was refreshed in the cool water. The cobra on Mr. G. rose to full height, opened its mouth, and flared its hood, his forked tongue ready to catch the geckos on our palapa ceiling.

The waves on Jeanne's hips came alive, and her koi would have swum away had she not kept her hand on it as she dove into the deep blue after her sunglasses. Her favorite cocktail, a martini, was tattooed on her arm, green olive and all. It runneth over, flowing into the ocean. The leopard spots on her leg matched the pillbox hat she wore to dinner. As we were eating, a man came up behind her and kept slapping her neck. He almost knocked her silly attempting to kill the big black spider that was tattooed there!

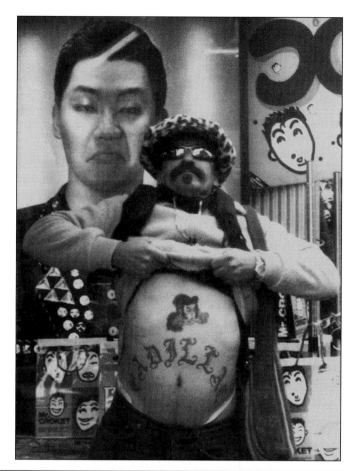

I could feel the slow burn of the sun on my back, roasting my Karmic Embrace tattoo. I'm sure I was the only woman along the entire east coast of Central and South America with such an image tattooed on her back. Remembering it was there, I immediately covered it up...the thought of death following me wherever I went and everyone seeing it... the sunburn I might get. Tattoos and vacations, ahh yes!

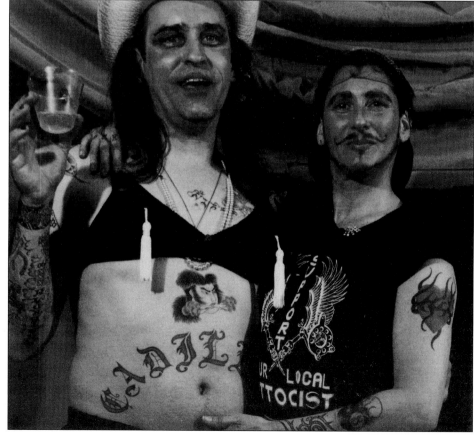

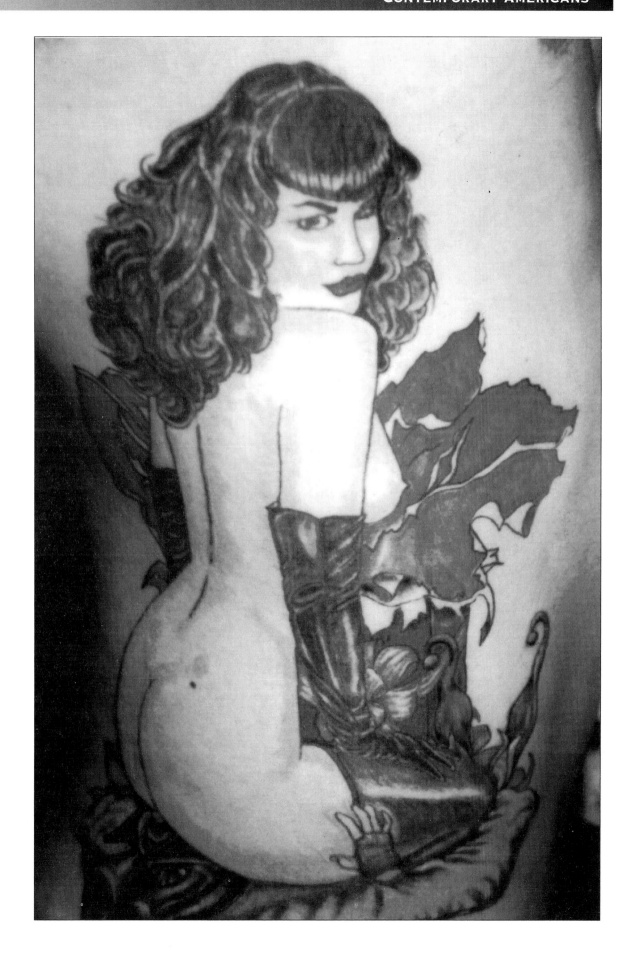

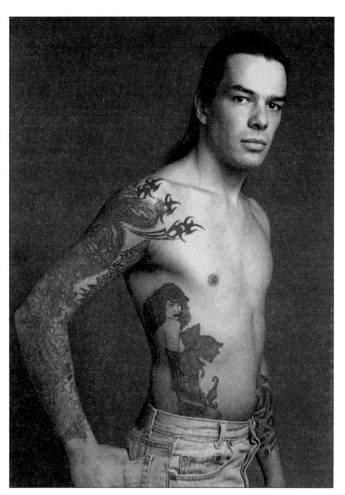

Dear Dad:

I dumped Susie, met a girl named Betty. She was hanging around at the tattoo studio. All she wears is red high heels. She is just a doll. She clings to my side like an ornament on a hot car. She doesn't say much. I like it that way. I've been sleeping with her for three nights now. At first I was a bit sore, but I'm getting used to her. She will be hanging out with me forever at this point. She is just luscious. I think you will like her, but I doubt if Mom will.
Love,
Shawn

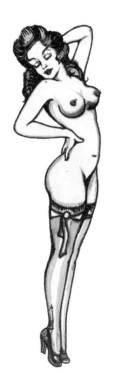

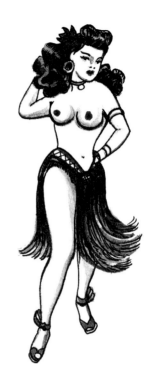

MEN'S CHOICES of tattoos differ from women's. One will rarely see a tattooed portrait of a man on a woman's body, while thousands of men sport tattoos of sexy women on their flesh.

I'll never forget the day a young man walked in the door clutching a photo of his wife in a bathing suit. He handed it to Mr. G. and asked, "Can you tattoo this picture of my wife on my arm, only I want her tits a little bigger and her waist a bit smaller?" With, tattoos men have the freedom to choose what their mates look like; her eye color, lip color, body proportions, everything. Most of these women have large perfect breasts with rosy nipples. They can choose whether she is clothed or naked, what position her body is in, and whether she is looking straight ahead, or if her eyes are demurely downcast.

The images of women that adorn the muscular arms of men worldwide are lofty, pink- skinned naked angels, Indian maidens with open rawhide shirts, Barbaric Trojan women draped in animal skins, and pin-ups, such as Betty Page, winged mermaid's, Goddesses, or pirate women bearing large swords with a patch over one eye. Portraits of Marilyn Monroe are found smiling out from the arms of more than a few men. Betty Boop is also popular. One young man settled for the words Girls! Girls! Girls! across his muscular freckled arm. A man from Germany who loves the sea, has his water bride, Pacifica, a mermaid, tattooed on his leg with a water dragon wrapped around her green-scaled body.

These images are married to their wearer. These silent luscious women will be the easiest and perhaps the most enduring relationship they will ever have.

THE HUMAN BODY: THE TATTOO ARTIST'S CANVAS

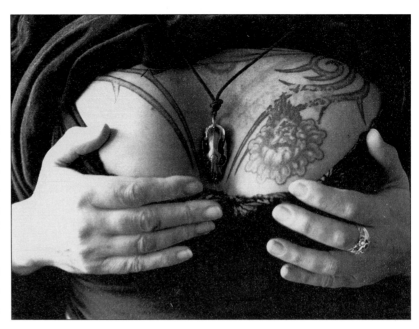

THE HUMAN SKIN IS a curious and exciting medium on which to create a design. It is unlike any other medium in the arts, because the life force behind this particular canvas has the freedom to act on the primitive urge by choosing to be marked with the image of their preference. The owner of this living, breathing, pulsing canvas will speak to us about their choice of a tattoo and their reasons for it. They must, also unlike other canvases or materials for the expression of art, seek their own design and the artist to tattoo it. This particular canvas has the innate realization that the mark they choose will be with them for life as an expression of their individuality.

As a canvas, human beings feel and express feelings of apprehension, fear, irritation, relief. And they will always leave with a distinct feeling of stunned exaltation. They will feel "lit."

Tattooing is an intimate art form. There is a synergetic connection between the artist and his or her canvas. The tattoo artist is a facilitator between the person being tattooed and their tattoo request. The relationship is many-faceted, psychological, spiritual, medical, philosophical as well as a technical, creative process.

The physical characteristics of human skin are unlike any other canvas in the artist's experience. It varies with each individual in texture, color, and temperament. It will puff up with histamines, flood with endorphines, bleed a bit with the abrasive process of getting a tattoo. It may rebel by flinching with involuntary muscle contractions. It may sweat. The skin's owner may faint, complain, bring the artists a flower, candy, take them to lunch, or write a bad check. These responses are different than any other medium because they pertain to a live canvas.

Tattooing is an intense media for the expression and act of art. It requires total cooperation between the artist and the human canvas. Like a prayer, it is a ritualistic process; like a dance, it requires two people with precise footing. It is a short-term relationship with lasting results. Utter self-confidence, expertise and incredible nerve are a necessary for this act of art. Once a line is tattooed under the skin, it is there to stay. There is no turning back, no possibility of erasure. There is an incredible edge to working with this wonderful and challenging medium.

Tattooing, like any art form, is a meditative act. It requires a point of reference and focus. The tattoo artist and his or her canvas becomes the very point of the needle that is being pushed under the third layer of skin at 2200 times per minute.

The owner of this canvas, unlike any other, commits to a selfish and enduring act. This necessitates strength of character and determination. It is an intense and enhancing experience. There is a significant and fundamental integration of the ink with flesh, the image with self. The human form is delightful to embellish. The natural contours of the body differ from person to person and are a challenge and pleasure to pursue in this artistic experience.

Tattooing has been a global art form, statement, and act for centuries. There is no canvas more sensual, more beautiful, more intriguing than the tattooed human skin.

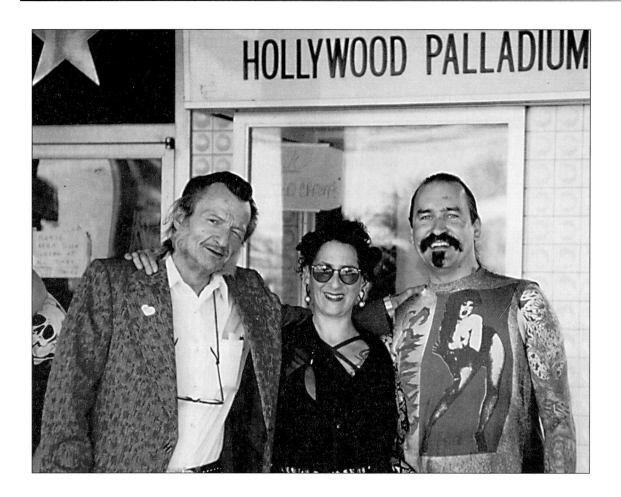

CONVENTIONS!

CONVENTIONS! THE WHITE NOISE, the profuse images and colors: The Bizarre. The Beauteous. The Macabre. It was all there… a continuous EYEGASM, pulsing under one roof. A roomful of common people raised to a magnificent level, strutting peacock-like with their tattoos. There was the steady beat of music, the incessant buzz of tattoo machines and the hum of conversations. Photographers swooped like vampires upon their subjects, stealing their souls with the blinding flash of the strobe light. So Intense!

Conventions are an occasion to mix with cohorts, see and show tattoos, enter tattoo contests, go to seminars and collect a tattoo as a momento of the event. It is also an opportunity to be photographed, interviewed, and communicate on like-minded subjects. We did all of the above.

Conventions draw people and artists from every walk of life worldwide. The attire is provocative; ovals

and designs are cut out of clothing to show-off tattoos. The tattooed person is never truly naked, being clothed in inked images.

Tribal designs contour muscular and voluptuous bodies. Wild felines crawl through jungle flora across smooth backs towards their prey. Realistic portraits of lovers, children or the deceased stare in a fixed state out from the skin of one who honors their memory. A dragon crawls across the belly of a woman who says it is "Ink For Her Soul."

Mona Lisa is alive and well on the freckled back of J. Scalrini. Dueling octopi write on a bony rib-cage, dolphins are at play in aqua blue waters across a man's corpulent stomach.

Dragons, winged horses, fairies, angels, mermaids, wizards, vikings and the like, are given life through the act of tattoo. We embody cultural and historical myths through this ancient art form. As this winged creature stares out from her pale white back, his steel blue eyes speak to us of ancient times, of cold stone walls in castles, of ethereal mists that rise dreamlike from moats, alligators snapping the cold night air.

Tattoos encompass the elemental and the fierce. They are at the same time mysterious and erotic. They transcend cultural boundaries. American Indian totems breathe next to Monkey Gods and Buddha's. A Samurai will share the same space with an Indian Warrior.

Flowers of all colors and stages of growth adorn the bodies of men and women, enduring the frigid winter, static in space and time on their warm-blooded wearer. A lunar eclipse breathes timelessly. Birds are in midflight endlessly. Confederate flags blow in a constant wind. Elvis, Bob Marley, Hitler, James Dean, Marilyn Monroe and more stare out at us with eternal eyes.

In 1992 at the Amsterdam Tattoo Convention Mr. G. collected many souvenir tattoos: a psychedelic neck piece from Phillip Leu; the bold black letters AMSTERDAM from Dave Shore, a peony from Horiyoshi III, a Samoan piece from Petelo Sulu-Ape. The word HOLLYWOOD was tattooed around his elbow with blue spotlights beaming out from a colorful polluted sunset by Aaron Caine. The King Theo Jack tattooed a pair of lucky dice on my arm, one is all 5s and the other all 2s, so I will always be a winner. These were tattooed in Hollywood at the Palladium in 1993. Last September at the Chicago Convention Mr. G., Sailor Cam and Calamity Jane got Buddy Guy's signature tattooed on them for a rack of BBQ'ed ribs from Hanky Panky. At the Santa Rosa Tattoo and Blues in March of 1994 I got a Goldfield rose from Henry and his seven-year-old daughter Lydia.

Yes, name-dropping! It's all part of the Convention scene. The magazines were all there: Tattoo Ink, International Tattoo, Hanky Panky's Tattoo World, Skin Art and more. Their photographers — Bill De Michele, Richard Todd, Deirdre Lamb, Wild Bill — were there recording the event.

Two years ago I was standing in the Hollywood Palladium, amidst hundreds of tattooed people taking it all in when I felt a gentle tap on my shoulder: "Hello, my name is Bill DeMichele." a man said to me. "I have the booth over there selling my first edition of Tattooed

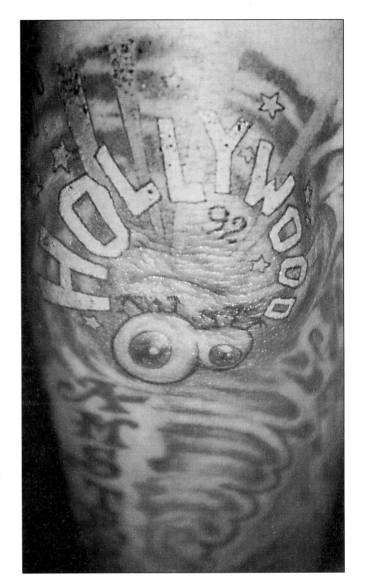

Women, and I would like to photograph you for my second. Next thing I knew, I was standing in front of a big sheet of paper in a small dark room with this stranger. I was hiding meekly behind the large black silk scarf which I had brought, consenting to drop it for three rolls of film... perhaps I will be one of the many tattooed women he has photographed in his second edition.

It is always a relief to return to the quiet of our home and comfort of our own bed. We are usually exhausted from over-stimulation of our senses and soothing the sting of a new tattoo. It is times like this when we don't care if we ever see another tattooed person again. At least... not until our noon appointments on Monday!

ARTISTIC MIXED MEDIA EXPRESSION

HOW OFTEN WILL ONE MEET an artist who is so committed to their art that they are compelled to have that image tattooed indelibly under the third layer of their skin? We know several! Point Richmond Conceptual artist Nicolino, creator of the Bras Across The Grand Canyon Project and Crazy Jimmy Pops are just a couple of them…

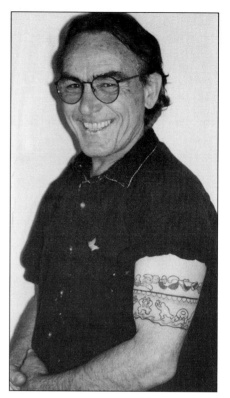

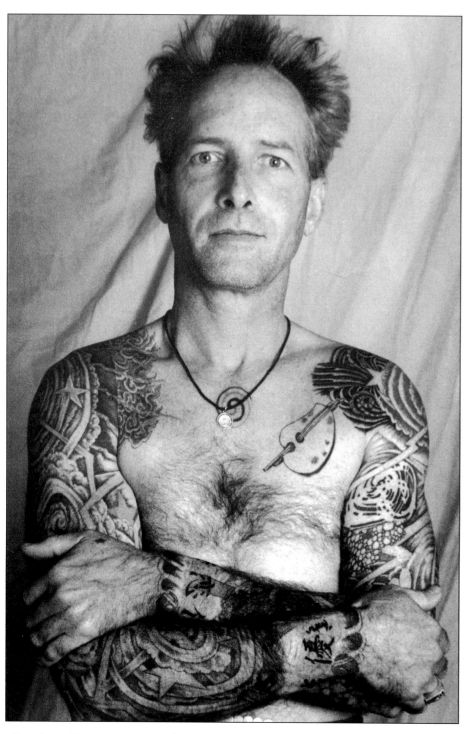

"These tattoos are talismans for the Bras Across The Grand Canyon project. They are two of three planned tribal totemic bands, representing significant stages in the process for completion of this odyssey. This totem pole arm insures my passage into the next world."

—attribution (Nicolino)

Crazy Jimmy Pops is a sign painter who wears his palette over his heart.

HERSTORY

THE TATTOOED WOMAN used to live in stone caves, under animal skin shelters, in igloos, mud-packed dwellings and under palm-thatched huts. She crouched near fire-pits collecting inky-black soot for her tattoos. She roamed naked and barefoot, proud and fearless upon the earth, collecting red berries and roots to grind into paste to tattoo herself. She would bow to the four directions — an elemental vibration resounding through the centuries. She was the Goddess, the Medicine Woman, the Woman of Pleasure, the Worker. She was the Mother.

Missionaries trespassed her lands, and shamed her into covering her nakedness, cutting her hair, and not praying to her animist gods. They shamed her into ceasing her "pagan ways," and marking her body with tattoos. She chewed strong roots and chanted while undergoing the tribal ritual of being tattooed for her passage into womanhood. She hid her tattoos behind black veils, silenced her tongue, but her soul was wild as ever.

She was tattooed by the Shaman or Tribal Elder, with sharpened obsidian, bones, fish teeth or metal. Ritual drums and chanting laced the night air. She was marked with symbols referring to her function in the tribe; as a basket maker, storyteller, medicine woman. She was marked when she was twelve and her menses began to flow, and again when they ceased.

In Gujarat, India, women were tattooed with vermilion inked dots at the corners of their eyes and face. Vermilion is the color of blood, and of the flames which will consume her body after death. Her tattoos were a rite of passage securing her safe journey into the afterworld amongst the wandering tribes.

In the fifties the tattooed woman was brazen, rebellious — often drunk and rowdy. She lingered in smoky bars with her tattooed shoulder exposed, and rode on the back of Harleys with her leather-encased legs clasped tightly around her man's hips. She smoked cigarettes, and drank beer, whiskey and wine, and still does. Her laughter echoes the centuries of her oppression. Her body dances the dance of all women in the slow and sensual undulations, in dusky atmospheres. She sucks from life urgently, like it's going out of style.

The tattooed woman may be seen sitting demurely on a high stool in a night club, crossing one slim ankle over the other, a tattoo barely visible through her dark silk stockings. She may be seen wearing a tattoo where her breast used to be. She can be seen lingering in static poses on the covers of CDs and fashion magazines.

The tattooed woman lives in ghettos, condos, in the streets... sleeps on newspapers. She bathes in rivers and in claw-foot tubs, uses a hole in the ground or a bidet. She can be seen sitting behind a desk with a computer mouse at her command, pushing a broom across smooth wooden floors, or dropping the children off at daycare. She works in a bank, the fields or in a crumbling government building. She holds a scalpel, wrench, spatula, hammer, blowdryer or a tattoo machine. The tattooed woman's archetype is diverse. She is an artist, housewife, teacher or secretary. She is a Christian, Buddhist, Jew, Quaker or Hindu. She is a republican, democrat, socialist or an anarchist. She is a vegan or she is omnivorous.

She is the aroma of amber, Egyptian musk, jasmine, patchouli or Chanel. Her hair is braided, permed or shaved. It is blond, henna or purple and perfumed by woodsmoke or fragrant oils. She wears an orchid in her French twist. She wears moccasins, Converse hightops, high heels, or Birkenstocks. Her dress is leather, cotton, fur, hemp, silk or polyester. She wears black opals, raw pearls, rhinestones, or sea shells around her neck.

Her flame is vibrant. She swims within her soup of hormones. The magnetism of the moon pulls her psyche. She encompasses the universal truths of all women...in all centuries...in varied states of consciousness. She rides the waves of her life with difficulty and grace.

We are all part of the Tribe of Women, beautiful and empowered by our tattooed symbols. We wear an eclectic mix of universal marks which are bizarre, traditional, artistic and graceful. They are disturbing and curious. With a feeling of revelation, we are sisters, dancing through this fire of ancient rituals, richly embellished, transformed forever, back into our lovers' arms, carrying within our hearts, as well as under our tattooed skins, an exquisite sameness...back into the world.

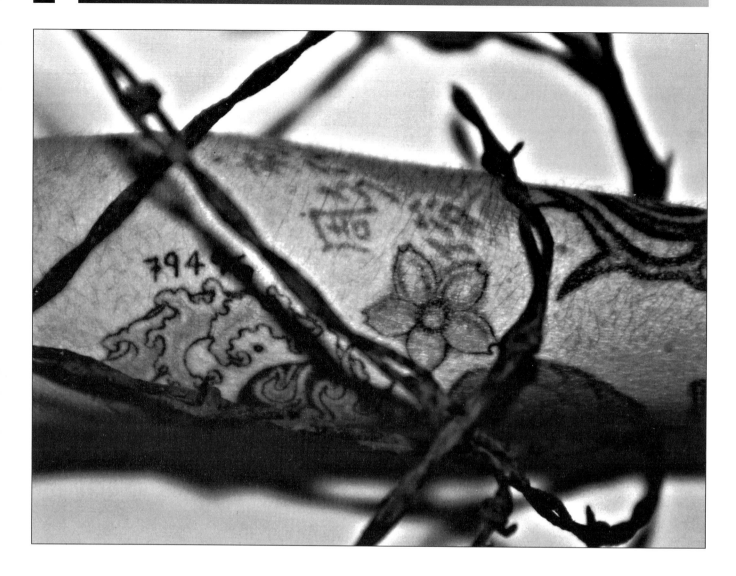

IN MEMORY TATTOOS: WE NAMED HER ROSE

"MY TATTOO SCREAMS THROUGH DECADES OF PAIN. It feels like a completion of someone who was never allowed to grow. It is my memorial, created out of respect, to all those people who survived or perished in Auschwitz."
– *Carol 1995*

"Without hesitation, I decided to have Chinchilla tattoo a tiny "Z" on my left shoulder, in memory of my unknown gypsy relatives who died in Auschwitz. All the gypsies were tattooed with a "Z" preceding their number (which stands for *zigeuner* which is German for gypsy). As she marked the letter in traditional blue ink, I thought about the pink triangles for gay men, black triangles for lesbians, yellow Stars of David for the Jews and the gypsies playing violin music in the camps…"
– *Francis Vavra 1995*

Historically, certain venerated symbols have been used as totems. These totems may be carved, sculpted, painted, woven or tattooed … ours are pushed under the third layer of our skins. On my own back, I wear a totem which I call the Karmic Embrace. It is a tattooed woman who represents me, embracing a skeleton. I also have the numbers 79496 tattooed in dark blue pigment on my left arm, and two cherry blossoms; all of which represent the fragility and transience of our lives.

In this century, we have few tribes or totems. Our rites of passage are being reinvented and reclaimed. Tribes have rituals for the passages of life. When a tribal member passes on in New Guinea natives smear their bodies with pig's fat and roll in ash. The Mayans would pierce their tongues, and other tribes worldwide wail.

As tattoo artists we have requests made of us which are varied and interesting. The words *Forever in My Heart, In*

Memory of Dad, and *Do Not Fade Away* are tattoos which often adorn the flesh to remember a loved one. Choosing an image associated with the loss of a loved one is a transcendental act. The memory will live on with each glance at this revered mark.

On my desk is an altar of sorts with crystals and incenses. Under the crystals are small pieces of paper with designs which are rich in significance. On these papers are various sizes of cherry blossoms. This is an "In Memory" tattoo, which I use as a ritual gift to the close friends of my dear friend Lynne Butler's son, Brian, who recently passed on. The cherry blossom signifies the fragility of life. The Samurais had these delicate blossoms drifting through their tattooed body suits as a symbol of their reverence for life. I have tattooed several of these cherry blossoms on Brian's friends. On Brian's 24th birthday, I tattooed an "In Memory" cherry blossom laced with Brian's ashes around his mother's umbilicus.

Also on my desk is a gray film container with a label "Annie's Dad's Ashes." Annie's father passed on several years ago and she decided to mix his ashes with colored pigments and have me tattoo them on her backpiece of a lotus and bamboo.

One busy Saturday there was a woman who felt she had to have a tattoo. When I first saw her she was standing in the main studio with her husband holding a small Japanese box in both hands in front of her, against her belly. When I asked her if I could help her with anything, she and her husband both started to cry. I took them into my studio. Through tears and sobbing she said to me, "I need a tattoo of a purple heart. I need it today. Please give it to me as soon as you can. Our baby died two days ago. These are her ashes. I had her by C-section. I want to be opened up and have her ashes put back inside of me, but that is unreasonable. We had to take her off of life support. We held her for two hours as she died. When we were driving home I was holding the ashes on my lap, and I saw your sign with the red hearts. I knew then that I need this tattoo."

By then I was crying with them and I rearranged appointments so I could tattoo a purple heart on her ankle. This was part of her healing process. We do many tattoos in our Main Street upstairs studio that are a ritual part of grieving and healing. There is an ancient feeling that goes on here when we are giving these tattoos to people.

I have an "In Memory" tattoo on my left arm. It is the numbers 79496. These are the numbers that were tattooed on a baby girl born in Birkenau on May 16, 1944. After several months of research for an exhibition for our Tattoo History Museum on *Tattoos Without Consent*, I received a contribution from the curator of the Museum of Tolerance from the Simon Weisenthal Center for Jewish Studies in Los Angeles. It was a copy of the diary of a tattooer who was at Auschwitz for two weeks in 1944. I came across the baby girl's number in the diary. On what would have been her 51st birthday I asked Mr. G. to tattoo her numbers in dark blue pigment on my arm. She was exterminated right after her birth. She was not given a name. No one heard the whisper of her name on her mother's lips as she was torn from her arms, taken away, and tattooed with the numbers I now wear on my arm.

Carol and I have chosen to wear the tattoo of her number, carrying with us — under our skins — her memory. This child shared the same birthday as Carol and the same religion as us both. On the day I tattooed the numbers 79496 on Carol, as part of the ritual I handed her a fresh red rose from my rooftop garden to hold. Before the tattoo needles pierced her skin, she said to me, "Wait! Let's give this baby girl a name." I looked at her and at the lovely red rose and said, "Let's call her Rose."

This young baby could have been me. I consider her my sister. These people — my people — were not given a printed instruction sheet on how to care for their new tattoos, so I did not take proper care of this tattoo. I did not carefully moisturize it and keep it out of the sun for two weeks. It is still there on my arm. The numbers are still on the arms of the Holocaust survivors. Carol and I have this tattoo in memory of that baby girl born on May 16, 1944 and in memory of all of the Jewish people who perished in WWII.

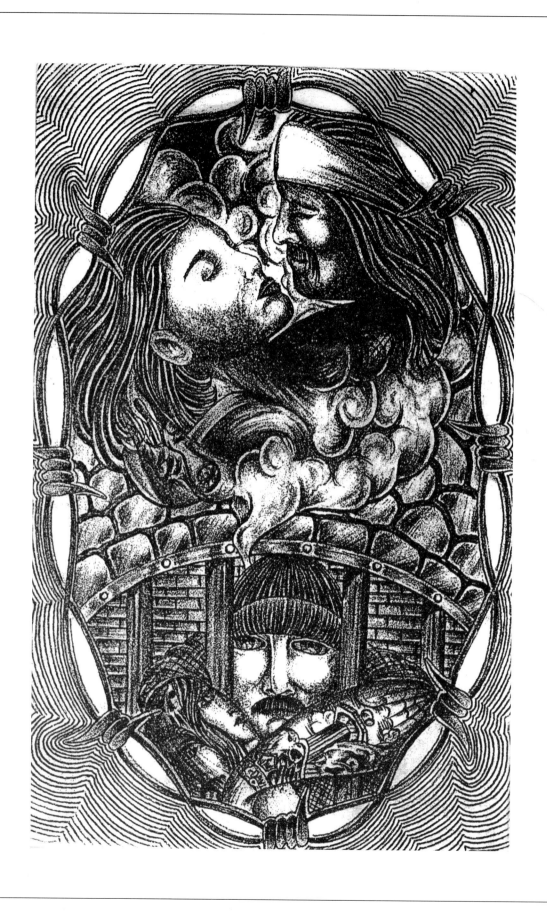

PRISON TATTOOS

PRISON TATTOOS ARE EARNED. They do not evolve from a whim. In Russia, they often match crimes. The tattoos an inmate wears show his status in the hierarchy which exists behind bars. To the inmate tattoos are something that cannot be taken away from them.

"I was mad at the world, rebellious when I got my tattoos, committed crimes and was in prison. I feel differently now. I have been out for three years and intend to stay out. The air smells so good out here. The colors of nature so brilliant. I will never go back to the cold steel atmosphere of prison. The town I live in and my job are my band-aid, and my woman, she is my angel. I feel good here and now."

— Dan

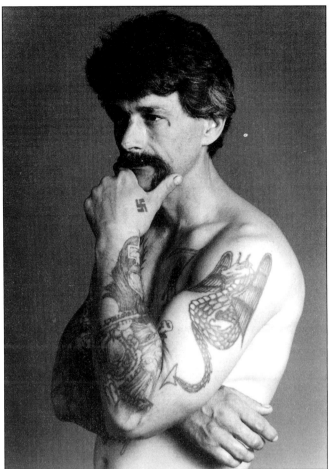

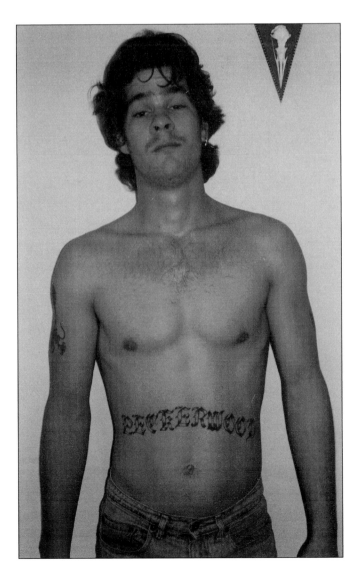

"In this life, someone can take everything we have, our clothes, home and family. They can make us lose our pride, our minds and our will power. They can lock us up. But these tattoos are mine. They will have to skin me to get them."

— Unknown inmate

The tattoos are done with prison guns made from walkman cassette players. Guitar strings are the needles and they are run by batteries. The tattoo pigment is made from a variety of things, burnt bible ash, Mr. Goodbar wrappers, toilet paper ash, burnt dominoes and shoe polish are just a few of them.

Self-expression is a necessity in the stark restrictive atmosphere of cold prison walls.

Sentimental art and tattoos are common amongst those who have loved ones waiting for them. Expressions of love, loneliness, anger, frustration, group security and identification are evident in prison art and tattoos. Tattooing is called LOCKED DOWN INK. It is illegal in prisons and done in secret.

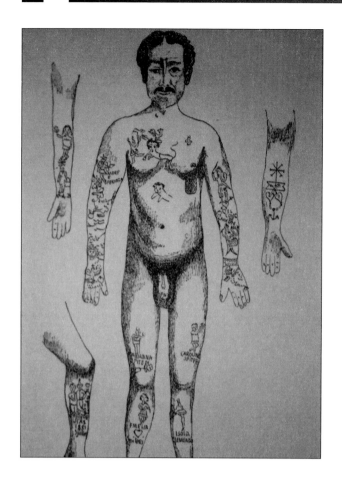
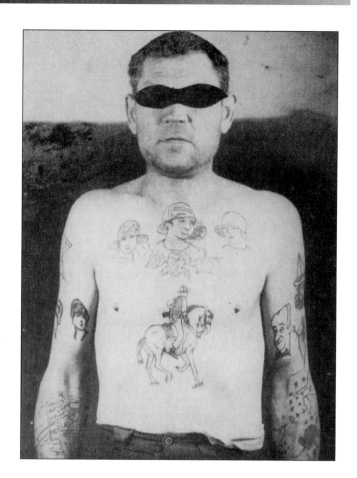
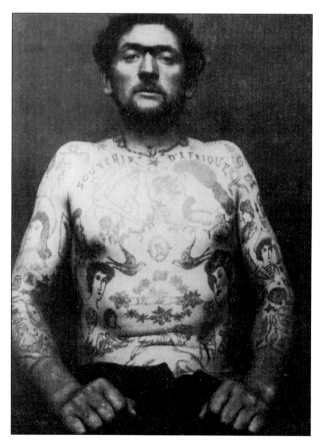
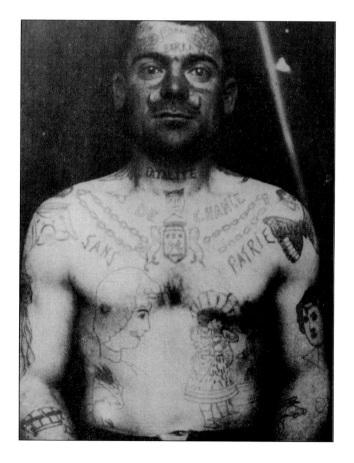

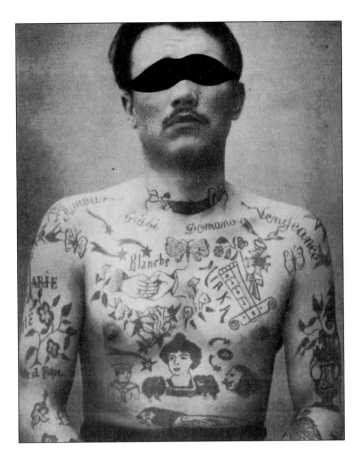
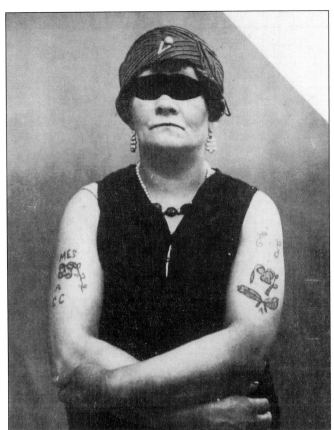
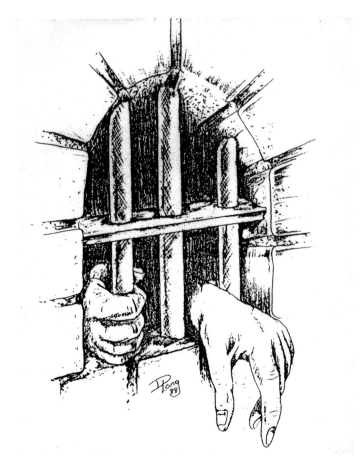

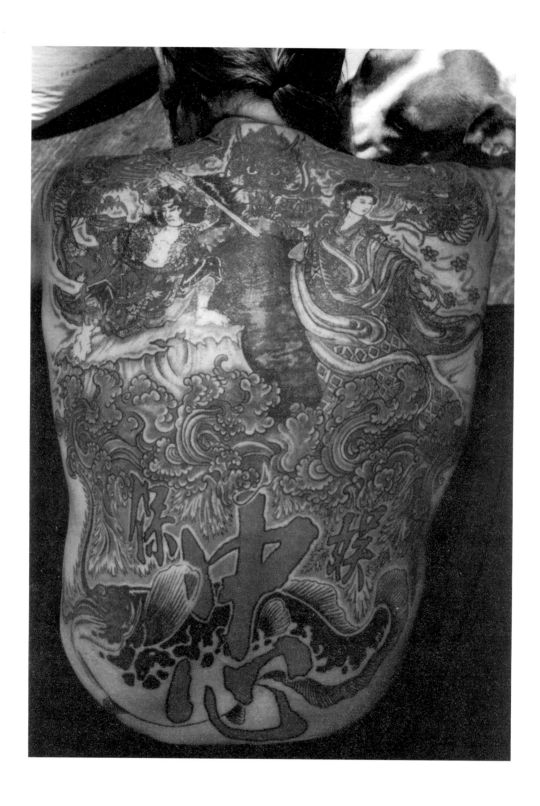

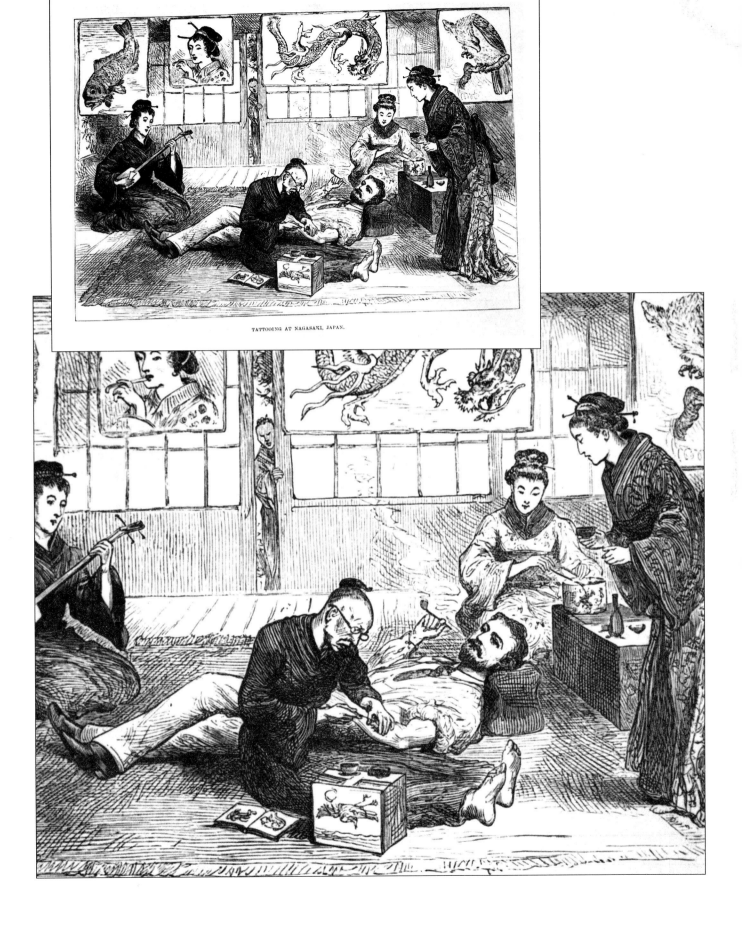

TATTOOING AT NAGASAKI, JAPAN.

SPIRIT OF JAPANESE TATTOOS

AS I SIT HERE ON THE NORTHERN COAST of California on this rainy morning, staring out our rooftop window, waiting for the coffee water to boil, I drift back into Horitoshi's studio in Ikabukuro, Japan. The memory of images devastates me. So brutal were the scenes etched under the smooth white skin of these young men. So powerful... The Samurai holding the severed head of another. His sharp metal sword

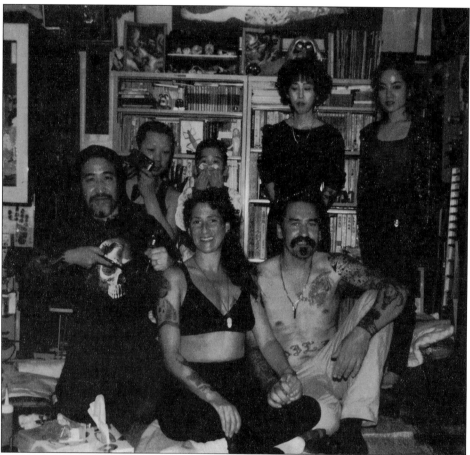

bloodied with its victory, an ominous gleam of satisfaction in the victor's dark eye.

I recall sitting primly in the studio of Horitoshi I, with Mr. G. The wintry wind howled outside the steamy windows, our legs were tucked under us, cramping, on the thick tatami mats. We were surrounded by eight curious men, each wearing tattooed body suits in various states of completion. A large bowl of gigantic strawberries and canned cold espresso were laid in front of us on a small lacquered table.

Looking back upon the scene of these creations, I

cringe when I remember the implements used to tattoo these monumental body suits. I have a vivid memory of sitting there, wide-eyed, gazing apprehensively at the metal rod, that had thirty-six steel needles bound to it like a concubine with red silken threads, knowing I was next in line to experience the sensations that bound these men to one another and to their culture. They endured arduous hours of these needles being maneuvered by hand after being dipped in black sumi ink, which was ground by hand by Ichuro, Horitoshi's son, his apprentice.

Japanese tattoo designs are mythical scenes on a grand scale. They are expressed in combinations of images, all meaningful and powerful. They are of wind and lightning, fire and water, swirling vortexes, drifting cherry blossoms, dragons, carps, and deities. They represent Life, Death, War, Wisdom, Serenity, Prayer, Transcendence, Beauty, Bravery, Devotion, Endurance, and Grace. Each tattoo is a perfect haiku, its beauty and passion, astonishing. The tattooed people in Japan associate amongst a nakarna (discreet group) of people. Their artists are unavailable to the general public. Only by special arrangement can one obtain entrance into their studios.

We met Horitoshi I and Horiyoshi III in Amsterdam at a tattoo convention where we received our first tattoos from them, and made arrangements to have another tattoo done in Japan. When we got to Japan, Mr. G. had a Samurai tattooed on his stomach (it looks like a Japanese Elvis), and I got a mythical snake with an orb between its razor-sharp teeth containing the symbol of my birth, which means "As Elusive As Lightning." In keeping with tradition, our tattoos were signed by the artist in a block.

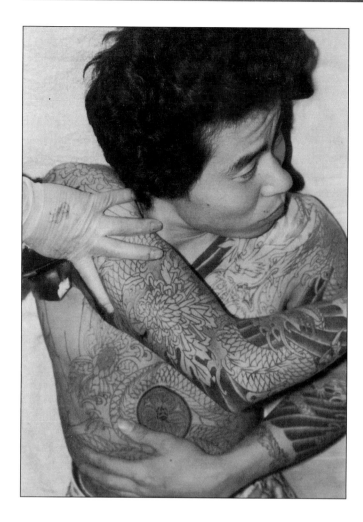

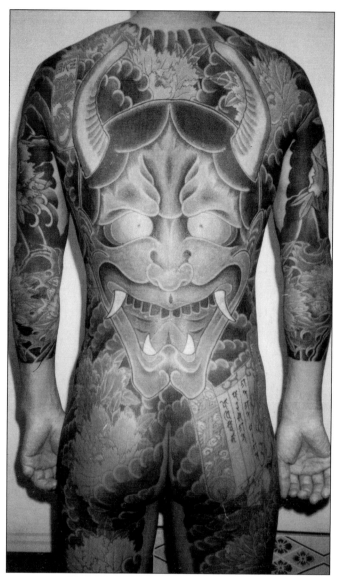

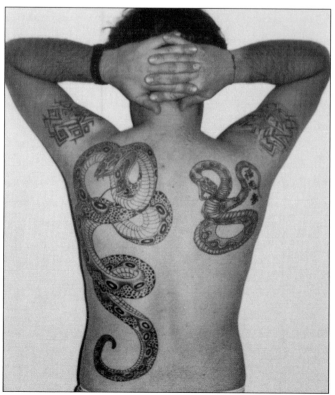

Japanese tattoos contain recurring themes of cherry blossoms, both on the branch in full bloom, and drifting, petal by petal, across the body, usually with wind behind them. These are worn by the Samurai and the courtesans as personal insignias indicating their recognition of the evanescence of their lives. Their flesh is as fragile as the petals of this delicate blossom. The chrysanthemum represents steadfastness, and the peony symbolizes wealth and good fortune. Also worn is the dragon, which combines the elements of fire and water and is often breathing flames. This mythological creature symbolizes the yin-yang and wholeness. He is often clutching an orb, which is believed to contain the spiritual essence of the universe. It is with this orb that he controls the movements of the wind, rains and planets. Everything about the dragon suggests power. His stance suggests natural energy.

Some of the deities used as tattoo themes are: Fudo; a fanged God of Wrath and Guardian of Hell, Kintaro, the carp Boy, Kannon, and Gagoroma; the goddess symbolizing compassion and understanding. They are from kimono designs and Noh plays. Tamatori-hime, another mythical image, a bare breasted diving girl provocatively playing with a dragon.

This iconography encompasses legends and myths of a complex, rigid, and curious culture. With part of their culture living under our flesh, we can be a catalyst and conduit to others. The possibilities are endless, until our living canvas is covered. So elemental and fierce was the feel of the sumi ink being pushed under this delicate flesh of mine. An elixir so brilliant... the mythical snake with the turquoise orb... illusive... the calligraphy, like a whisper in the northwesterly wind... oh... gotta go now... water's boiling!

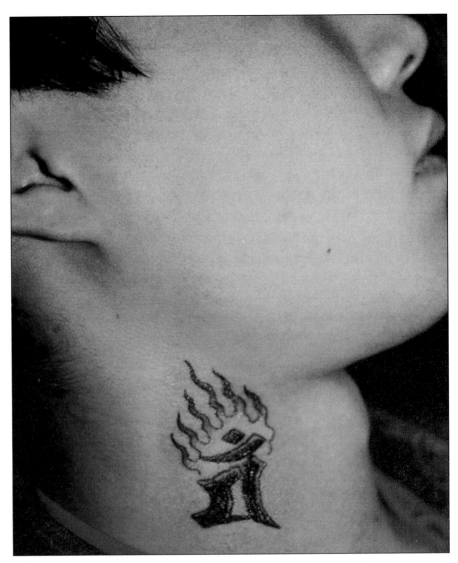

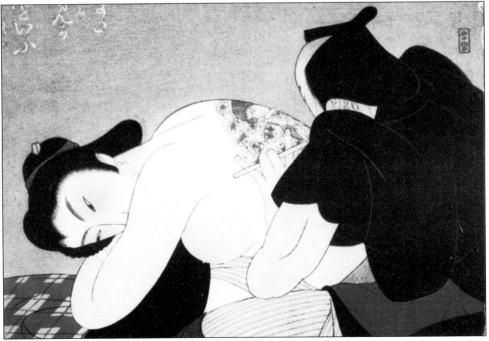

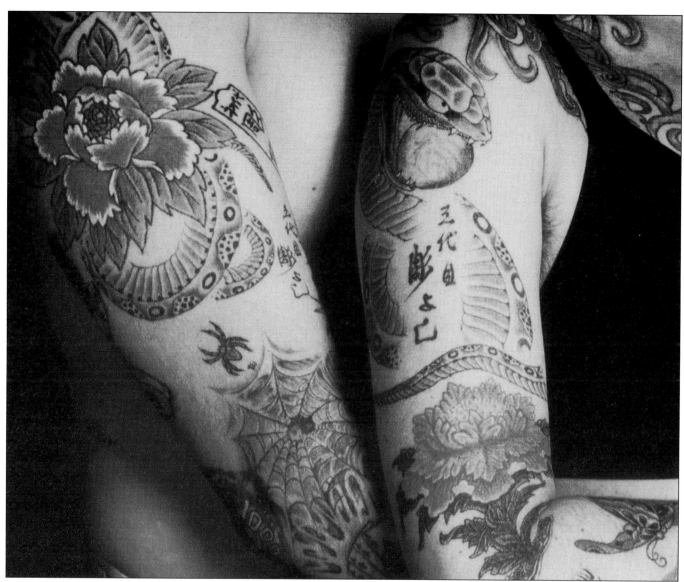

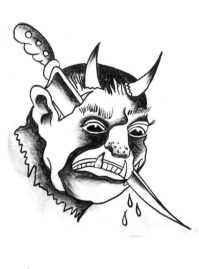

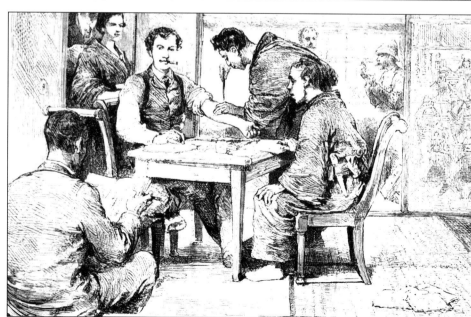

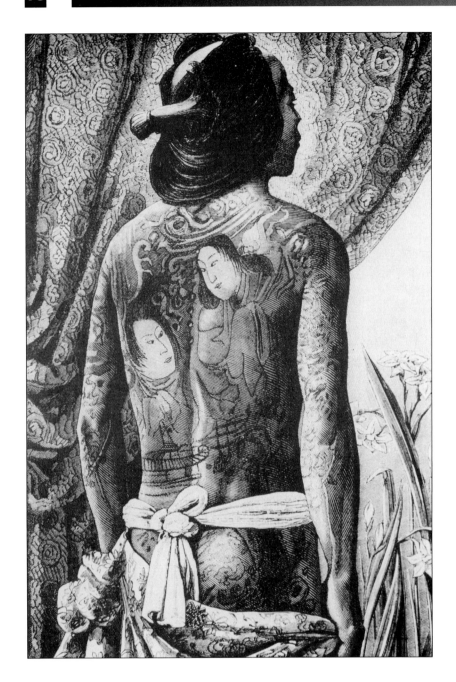

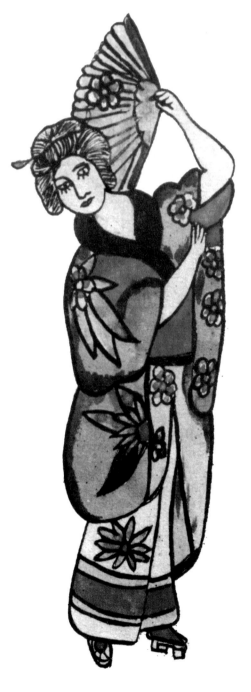

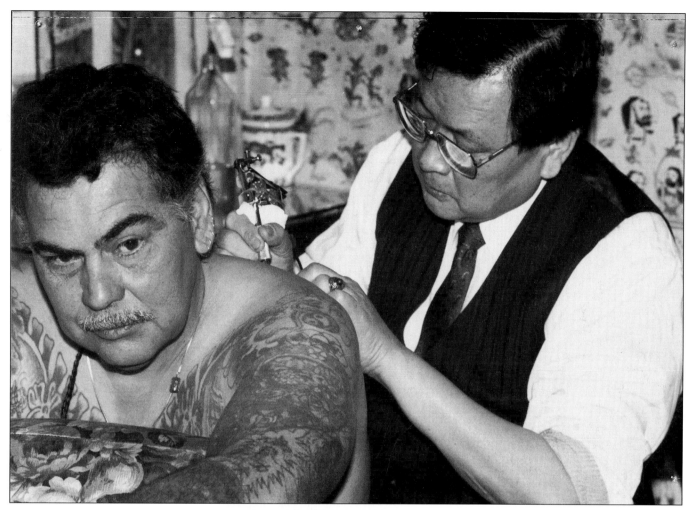

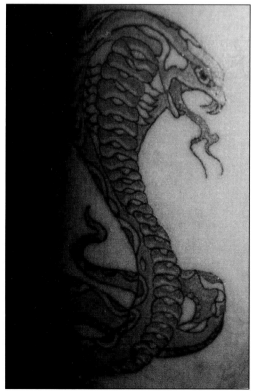

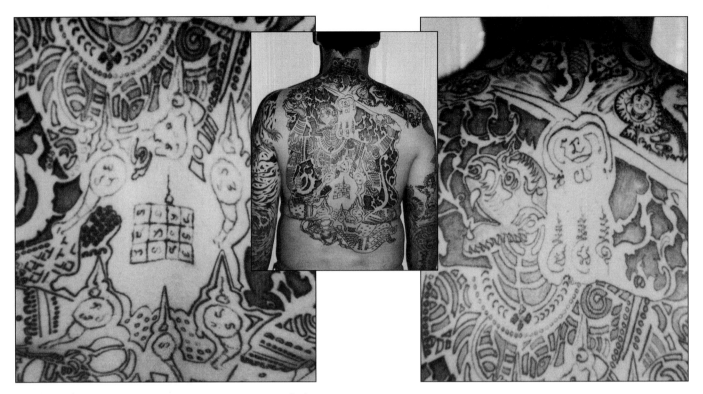

MR. G.'S YANTRA NORTHERN THAILAND

"Holy and beneficial tattoos are called Yantras. These markings are so powerful that the person who wears them is considered under divine protection. A sword can be pressed against the tattooed spot and it will not penetrate the flesh."

— *(but, Mr. G. has not tried that yet.)*

WE PROPELLED OURSELVES ACROSS the Great Pacific Ocean, and overland to the Wat Kumparadit in Northern Thailand, in quest of Sandom Sakom, the only Monk who performs Yantras. We stayed four days with this powerful man, absorbing the flavor, rituals and prayers he exuded.

A heavy rain was falling — the air was thick and sweet with temple incense. We felt a quiet lethargy. It was at this time that Mr. G. asked for a Yantra. Sandom Sakorn looked deep into his eyes and nodded his bald, shiny head, yes. He reached into a large, black lacquered bowl containing his tools. First, he withdrew a bottle containing a mixture of flower petals, sacred oil, amulets and other magical elements. Then he assembled the instrument for tattooing – a brass rod 2" long consisting of three parts screwed together, with a brutal point and a split in the end to hold the oil. He started chanting, breathing and moving his hands in a significant manner. He used his breath to blow the prayers into the atmosphere, and into Mr. G. who was

sitting with his shirt off, his chest bare except for the tiger head spewing forth the prayer Om Padme Hum. Arched across his stomach were 2-inch-high Old English letters spelling "CADILLAC." His legs were politely tucked under him, cramping, feet pointed away from Sandom.

He was in a state of pained ecstasy, as Sandom repeatedly drove this instrument into his chest, creating fifteen puncture marks. Tears were streaming down his cheeks, blood was seeping from these marks, done with sacred oil. They would leave no visible mark other than a slight raising of the skin. We were all affected by this ritual. The air was charged.

Sandom Sakorn sealed the prayers in with a small square of gold leaf, placing one on each puncture and rubbing it into him with sacred oil until it left a fine glittering effect. He did the same with his third eye, on each temple and into the palm of each of his hands, all the while chanting, praying and breathing these prayers into him.

Monks are not allowed to touch women, so he gave me a divine protective prayer with Mr. G. performing the rites. Glittering with gold leaf and infused with prayers we were enriched like a garden with black loamy soil, blooming roses and leafy bamboo.

HOUY KUNG VILLAGE NORTHERN THAILAND

WHEN KRITTONG KHAMLAUNGWAN pushed the sacred oil mixed with black, sooty pigment under Mr. G.'s skin, we tapped into a whirlpool of ancient energy. It was well past midnight but it was timeless as an opium dream. This Aztec-looking man, a Burmese ex-monk, now a shaman, walked to this village to tattoo us. He chanted prayers in the old Buddha tongue "Pali." They came in raspy whispers sounding like primitive secrets. A thin white candle flickered eerie light on Mr. G.'s tattooed back.

This tattoo experience was cosmic. The ritual connected us to a history written and recorded under the human flesh. This flesh is found mummified worldwide. The ink is like sap from the Tree of Life, and it connects us to the past, our roots... we can feel it.

The tattoo images were powerful and became even more so as he inked them into Mr. G.'s back. TIGER ENERGY... MAGIC... our translator told us.

Magic is curious... . It is translated as a *Mysterious Quality of Enchantment*. It comes in many forms. It can be encapsulated in a crystal or a piece of sculpted metal. or chanted in the breath of various tongues, it can also be pushed under the flesh with ink. It exists in all the elements: EARTH... WIND... FIRE... WATER. It is communicated with symbols expressed with sacred pigments, with sandalwood burning on joss sticks on wondrous nights in the jungle... surrounded by the shadows cast on bamboo walls by the last candle.

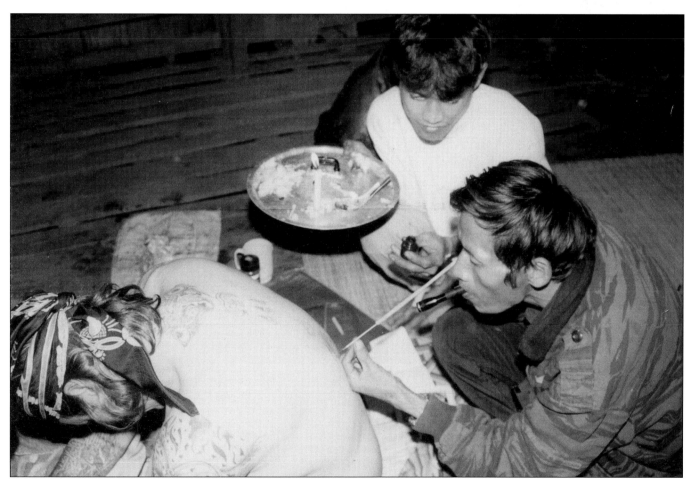

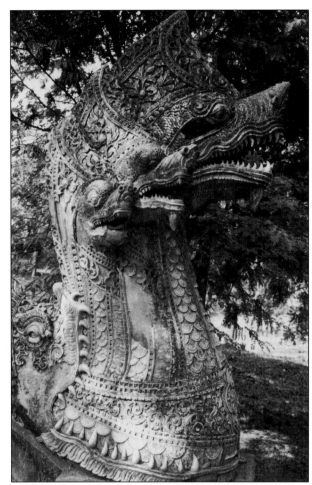

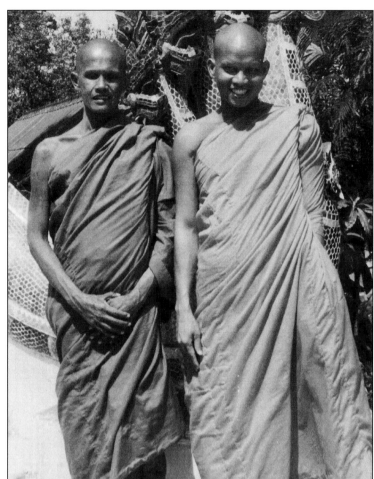

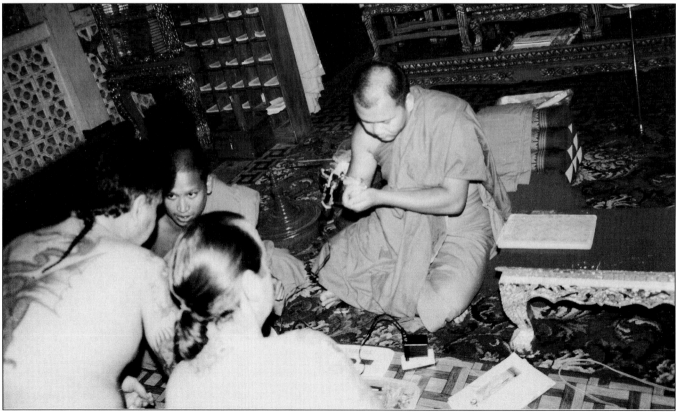

EAST MEETS WEST

SWEET SMOKE FROM TEMPLE incense mists the mid-day air. We are sitting on a hard mahogany floor with our legs tucked uncomfortably under us, our feet pointed away from Sankom Sakom, the Monk Tattooist. He is sitting in his opulent altar surrounded by Buddha figures.

His tattoos seem shy, peeking out from his saffron robe; garudas, tigers and religious calligraphy are red welted patterns on his skin. They are infused with ground red stone mixed with sacred oil. He also wears invisible images which are tattooed with sacred oil. They are for protection and magic.

These tattooed markings are hand-poked using a brass instrument with a brutal point that is kept in a large hand-painted lacquer bowl next to his sacred blends. He is a magnificent sight to behold, bearing the indelible marks of Buddha, his deity.

We are like monkeys with our curiosity, showing him our tattoos. He likes them very much, although he's not impressed with them on a religious, magical level. He especially likes the tattoo of the butterfly on my arm, points to it, and has our interpreter ask us if Bert Rodriguez will tattoo it on him. We trace the pattern from my arm and place it on his. He cannot touch me, as Monks cannot touch women. This is his first decorative tattoo, which he will

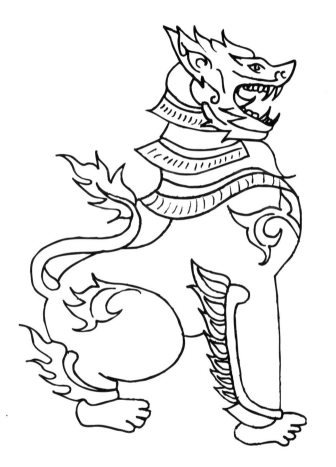

wear on his left arm, discreetly hidden under his saffron robe.

We hear chanting and insects clicking, along with the electric buzz of our tattoo machine which is pushing colorful ink under this Monk's golden flesh.

The butterfly is finished. He is rapt, and gazes at it as though it were a magical creature that had just landed there. This is a fine moment; we are all pleased. A colorful butterfly matching mine, now bonds us to this man. He brings out a tin of stale English cookies and instant coffee. We eat and drink together as a cool breeze blesses us like a prayer.

Like an elixir, this diverse mixture of beliefs and personal preferences lays under the third layer of our skins, like a praying mantis ready to spring forth in celebration of our new friendship.

It was under the spell of this intoxicating jungle atmosphere, just after a deluge of rain, when the smells rose up like a phoenix, spicy and exotic, that we received our yantras, and traded tattoo implements with the Monk. This was the day he stepped through centuries of tradition and received the tattoo of my butterfly, and this was the day that Sadom Sakom went electric. Yes… East met West in a profound moment that day in the Wat Kumparadit, a monastery in Northern Thailand.

WAT OF THE BIG BUDDHA S.E. THAILAND

LIKE FOOLISH TOURISTS we ventured out into the hellish hot noonday sun on a small motorbike (whose gears shift backwards), through steamy jungle roads to the Wat of the Big Buddha. The stunning sight of mythical temple guardians greeted us.

Emerald green dragons slithered up each side of the handrail leading up to a gigantic Buddha who sat in a state-

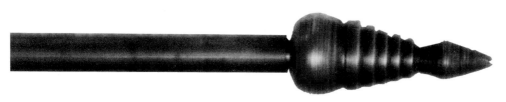

ly manner above the temple grounds overlooking the Sea of Siam. It was a religious experience standing there amongst so many surreal creatures. At the base of the stairway a typical tourist shopping area sold amulets, delicious food, water, sun-hats and various exotic yet common indigenous goodies. It was at this Wat that I saw the most profound tattooed statement in my life. On the sun-parched arm of a 55-year-old Buddhist Monk were the

words I DON'T CARE LADY with a heart and dagger. I asked our interpreter permission to photograph this Monk's tattoos, and as I was doing so his robe slid to the side and I discovered another tattoo of considerable interest on his thigh. It was a woman hanging on the underside of a horse, and copulating with it. Shocked and intrigued we stood there in a sweaty swoon from the immense heat, eating fried bananas, drinking cold coconut milk from the shell, and ogling at these incredible statements of a sexual nature on the Holy Man! He had tattoos on his hands, chest, and entire back legs and feet. Religious symbols, calligraphy and these two aforementioned tattoos made him a sight to behold as he stood there under an exotic tree with his ochre robe all askew in order to let us photograph his tattoos. A praying mantis was perched on his shoulder like a talisman. We asked our interpreter the meaning of these tattoos, and as far as we could understand the story was…

"As a young man and not yet a Monk, he lived in a

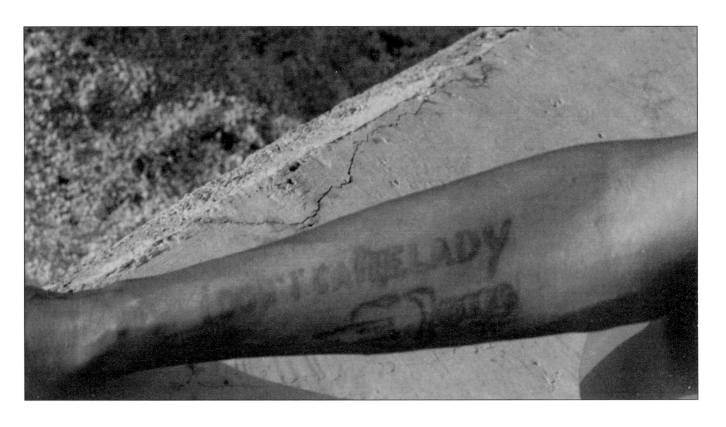

poor village in northern Thailand near the Burmese bor-der. It was common for the people to get decorative tat-toos, so he chose these to express his choice of celibacy and feelings about marriage. He had no dowry, and felt a sense of rejection so he marked himself in this manner and joined the Monastery at the age of 17, intending to remain…"

He was very pleasant. We visited him several times and taped him chanting. He asked for a photo of Mr. G. and me and our interpreter. On our last visit with him, we gave him a photo of us sitting with him which is now hanging on the wall at the Wat of the Big Buddha on a small tropical island floating like an emerald on the Sea of Siam. Despite our cultural differences, we followed the common thread through the Ancient Art of Tattoo to one another.

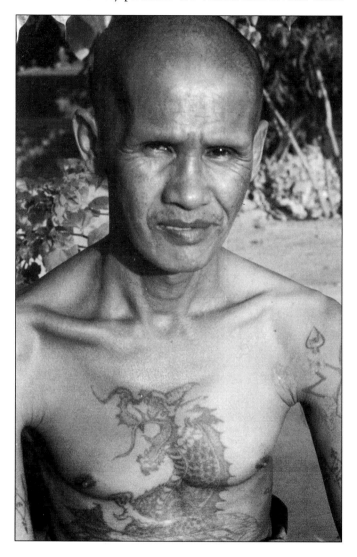

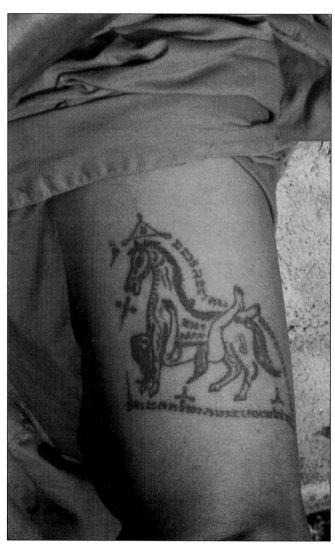

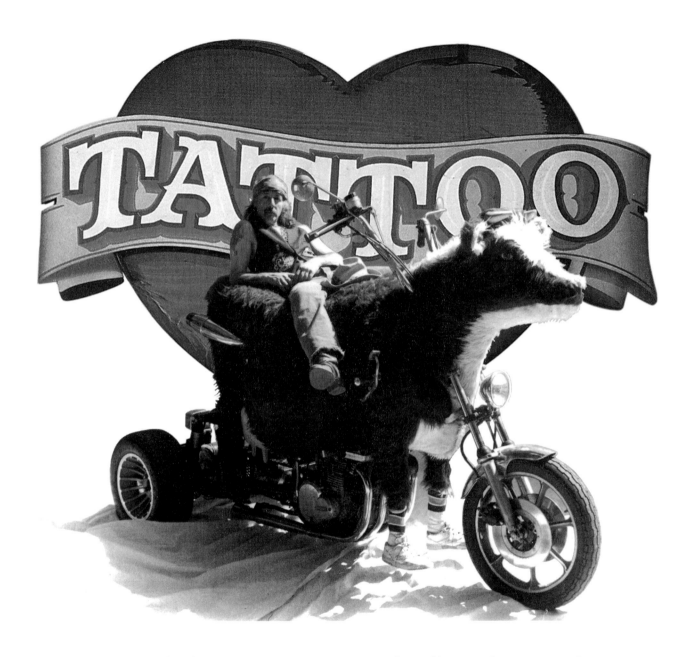

"As we travel life's highway, we cannot escape the effects of our socialization. Our role within various groups, and the decision to follow the norms of these groups, provide a map for our travels. Occasionally, whether consciously or not, we select an alternate route or a detour along the way. In a break from the ideal norms that surround me, the detour I chose took me to a tattoo parlor."

—— Kathy Chatwin

SELECTED BOOKS & OTHER RESOURCES

BOOKS:

Bad Boys and Tough Tattoos; A Social History of the Tattoo With Gangs in New York, Harrington Park Press, 1990.

How To Do Good Tattooing, Miss Cindy Ray, Australia, 1970.

Maori Tattoo, Ko Te Rivia, David Simmons, Bush Press, 1989.

Marks of Civilization, Arnold Ruben, Los Angeles Museum of Cultural History, UCLA, 1988.

Modern Primitives, Research #12, Vale V. & Andrea Juno, 1989.

Moko, Michael King, 1992.

Pierced Hearts & True Love, Hanns Ebensten, Shenual Press, 1953.

Pierced Hearts & True Love; A century of drawings for tattoos, The Drawing Center & Don Ed Hardy, 1987.

Polynesian Tattooing, Alan Taylor, Brigham Young University, Hawaii, 1981.

Sacred Calligraphy of the East, John Stevens, Shambala Press, 1995.

Sailor Jerry Collins; American Tattoo Master, Hardy Marks Publications, 1994.

Tatau, Chief Sielu Avea, Selu Enterprises, 1994.

Tattoo: Pigments of the Imagination, Alfred Van der Marck, New York, 1987.

Tattoo Times 1-5, Don Ed Hardy, 1987.

Tattooed Women, SkinShows, Chris Wroblewski, 1987-1995.

The Prison Experience, Morrie Camhi, Tuttle IPC, 1989.

The Tattoo Book, C.H. Fellowes, Master Tattooer, Pyne Press, 1971.

Total Tattoo Book, Amy Krakow, Warner Books, 1994.

RESOURCES:

Archive Files: Chuck Eldridge, 1986-1996.

"Tattoo Advocate," Shotsie Gorman, 1990.

"Tattoo Historian," Lyle Tuttle, 1982-1986.

"Tattoo International of Great Britain," Lionel Titchner, 1987-1996.

FUTURE PUBLICATIONS:
He Who Lives By the Sword Is Always Broke, Captain Don Leslie, Sword Swallower, Isadore Press, 1998.

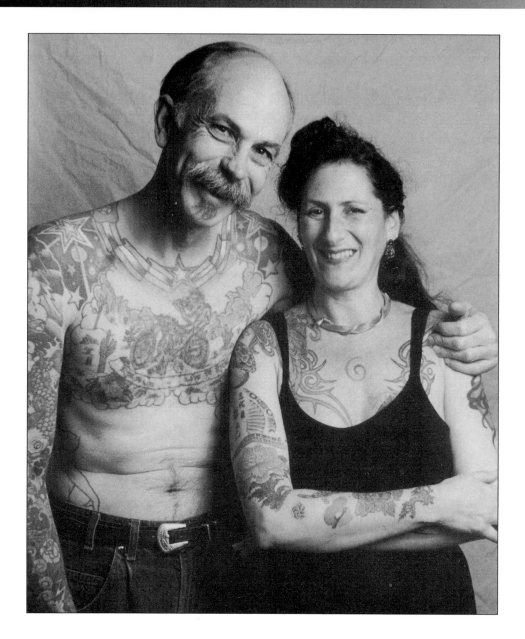

THE ARCHIVIST & THE AUTHOR

Madame Chinchilla is a Tattoo Artist and Museum Curator at Triangle Tattoo and Museum in Fort Bragg, California. She is a columnist for National Tattoo Association, Tattoo International of Great Britain, Tattoo Ink Magazine, The Mendonesian *(a local newspaper)*, and A.P.T. Her columns are titled SKINTALK. She has been published in numerous other publications.

C.W. Eldridge is a Tattoo Artist and Tattoo Historian in his Berkeley Tattoo Archive and Studio in Northern California. He provided archival material and support for this book. He is a lecturer on Tattoo History, has a mail order business of tattoo collectibles and is a Member of the Board of Directors of the Paul Roger Tattoo Research Center; as well as Historian for the National Tattoo Association. He is an avid bicyclist and loves sleeping late between flannel sheets.

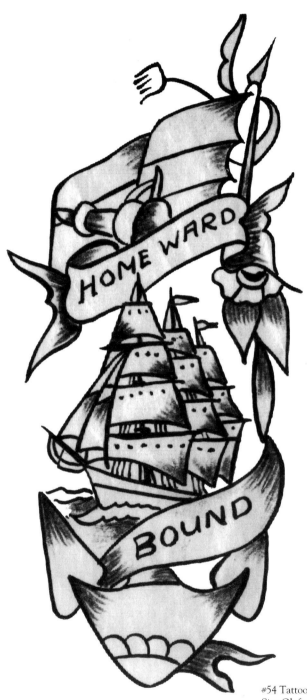

HOME WARD

BOUND

#54 Tattoo Peter Design
Sint Olofssteeg, Amsterdam

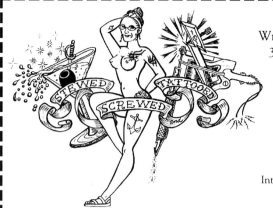

For Ordering Additional Copies

Write To: ISADORE PRESS, c/o Triangle Tattoo Museum
356B North Main Street, Fort Bragg, California 95437

Send your
Personal Check
US Postal Money
Order or
Bank Cashiers
Check Only

Please Send Me _____ Copies of
STEWED, SCREWED & TATTOOED

I have enclosed $20.00 for each copy ordered _____

Include $5.00 Shipping & Handling for each copy ordered _____

California Residents Please Add 7.25% Sales Tax _____

International Orders Will Be Shipped Airmail Please Add $10.00 Per Copy _____

Total Amount Enclosed _____

Discounts Are Available For
Large Orders, Please Inquire:
707 964-8814 or
FAX 707 964-6770

Available In The United Kingdom:
Tattoo Club of Great Britain
389 Cowley Road, Oxford, Great Britain

Available In Germany:
Tatowier Magazin, Ottenhofer StraBe 8
D-68239 Mannheim, Germany
TeleFax 06 21-48 361-74

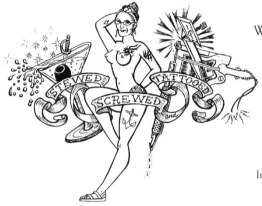

For Ordering Additional Copies

Write To: ISADORE PRESS, c/o Triangle Tattoo Museum
356B North Main Street, Fort Bragg, California 95437

Send your
Personal Check
US Postal Money
Order or
Bank Cashiers
Check Only

Please Send Me _____ Copies of
STEWED, SCREWED & TATTOOED

I have enclosed $20.00 for each copy ordered _____

Include $5.00 Shipping & Handling for each copy ordered _____

California Residents Please Add 7.25% Sales Tax _____

International Orders Will Be Shipped Airmail Please Add $10.00 Per Copy _____

Total Amount Enclosed _____

Discounts Are Available For
Large Orders, Please Inquire:
707 964-8814 or
FAX 707 964-6770

Available In The United Kingdom:
Tattoo Club of Great Britain
389 Cowley Road, Oxford, Great Britain

Available In Germany:
Tatowier Magazin, Ottenhofer StraBe 8
D-68239 Mannheim, Germany
TeleFax 06 21-48 361-74

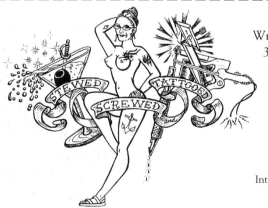

For Ordering Additional Copies

Write To: ISADORE PRESS, c/o Triangle Tattoo Museum
356B North Main Street, Fort Bragg, California 95437

Send your
Personal Check
US Postal Money
Order or
Bank Cashiers
Check Only

Please Send Me _____ Copies of
STEWED, SCREWED & TATTOOED

I have enclosed $20.00 for each copy ordered _____

Include $5.00 Shipping & Handling for each copy ordered _____

California Residents Please Add 7.25% Sales Tax _____

International Orders Will Be Shipped Airmail Please Add $10.00 Per Copy _____

Total Amount Enclosed _____

Discounts Are Available For
Large Orders, Please Inquire:
707 964-8814 or
FAX 707 964-6770

Available In The United Kingdom:
Tattoo Club of Great Britain
389 Cowley Road, Oxford, Great Britain

Available In Germany:
Tatowier Magazin, Ottenhofer StraBe 8
D-68239 Mannheim, Germany
TeleFax 06 21-48 361-74